The Natural Way to Stress Control

SIDNEY LECKER, M.D.

GROSSET & DUNLAP
PUBLISHERS • NEW YORK
A FILMWAYS COMPANY

To Della, the romantic
To Tammy, the treasure
To Wendy, the scholar
To Jamie, the lionhearted, with soul
To Stephanie, the child and Stephanie, the woman

Copyright © 1978 by Sidney Lecker, M.D.
All rights reserved.
Published simultaneously in Canada
Library of Congress catalog card number: 77-87787
ISBN 0-448-14539-1

Printed in the United States of America

Contents

Introduction

Every era has had its own unique set of problems which the inhabitants of the time must conquer in order to flourish or even survive. Throughout history, men and women have struggled against starvation and fear of the unknown. They tried to survive plagues against which there was no defense; and they were terrified by mental illness which was only understood in mystical or religious terms.

Twentieth-century science and technology pierced the veil of ignorance surrounding mental illness; antibiotics and vaccinations eliminated the threat of runaway epidemics; and fear of starvation gave way to a concern with self-actualization. This is an era of achievers and seekers — not satisfied to rest on its intellectual and technological laurels. We search for challenge, growth and positive change. Out of this national ambition has arisen a new epidemic — runaway stress problems.

The mental, physical and social manifestations of stress abound and preoccupy us — not as a deterrent to achievement but as an accepted part of life. We have begun to take it for granted that hard-working people will inevitably have heart attacks or ulcers; overly tense people rely on tranquilizers in growing numbers that reflect the major scope of the stress epidemic; and industries are beginning to arise specifically to help high achievers survive the onslaught of overwhelming stress that is generated in people by the culture of the post-industrial state. One such organization, E.H.E. STRESSCONTROL Systems, Inc., operates an institution in New York City called the STRESSCONTROL Center. I am one of the founders and the medical director of this organization.

In this book, I will explain the systems we use in coping with the stresses of high achieving executives. The techniques employed at our center are simple, easy-to-learn, effective solutions to the problems of stress. Mastery of stress control methods requires only that you learn the principles described in this book with a determination to implement these methods as a way of life. As contrasted with medical treatment, there is no magic in this stress control approach. You are your own "doctor" and must detect and relieve potentially harmful stress when it occurs and, ideally, even prevent its occurence when possible.

You may not be aware of it but I am certain you now intuitively use some effective stress control methods in your daily life. Making up a schedule to help you get through a hectic period at work distributes your finite energies effectively to important priorities — that's good stress control. The stress control system I have developed capitalizes on your natural reflexes in coping with stress, strengthened by some streamlined techniques developed by psychiatrists and psychologists who practice high impact short term psychotherapies. Among the individuals who have influenced my thinking and consequently whose philosophies are represented in the STRESSCONTROL program are: the late Dr. Maurice Levine, Dr. Nathan Epstein, Dr. Hyman Caplan and, of course, the various schools of psychiatry that have grown from the work of Sigmund Freud, particularly the ego psychologists. Special recognition must be given to the pioneering work of Dr. Hans Selye, who opened up the scientific frontiers concerning the study of stress. Single-handedly, he persisted for decades exploring this vital area until the world caught up.

The essence of the STRESSCONTROL System is action: action in retrieving information; action in processing that data; and an action-based approach to solving problems. The men and women whom we assist at the STRESSCONTROL Center want results in a reasonable time span — not indefinite delving into the past. Our methods complement, not replace or compete with, psychotherapy. What distinguishes them the most from traditional approaches is their speed, focus and action orientation.

The experience I have had as a psychiatrist in private practice and also in my work with corporate executives at the STRESSCONTROL Center in New York has convinced me that the difference between people who succumb to stress and those who effectively control it lies in the strategies employed when encountering a taxing situation. Time after time, when cases are reviewed and analyzed, a similar pattern emerges. The group that is more successful at controlling stress instinctively employs three stress management techniques:

1. Proper focusing on the source of the stress
2. Positive psychological rehearsal of effective coping methods
3. Implementation of solutions and preventive methods at times when stress occurs

Each person whom I counseled to control stress more effectively eventually had to learn these methods of coping, as they can be applied to stress in all of its manifestations. Some examples of small and major stresses are offered here to help illustrate these useful methods for keeping stress under control — making it work for you rather than against you.

Let's examine stress and how it affects memory, as an example. How many times have you had the experience of searching for a word which is on the tip of your tongue but not being able to retrieve it. The harder you concentrate trying to recall the word the more elusive it becomes. Finally, just as you give up and begin to turn your attention elsewhere, the word pops into your mind. What kept that word from appearing in your consciousness when you willed it so strongly to reveal itself? The answer is *stress* — or more particularly, the stress produced by the mental challenge of testing your memory and recall. You began to feel some stress by not having easy access to a word which was just out of reach. You intensified the stress by *improper focusing* and the net result was that the word became even more inaccessible.

What do I mean by improper focusing? Have you ever used a pair of binoculars at a football game or a camera with a zoom lens? You know, if you have, that when you want to focus to where the action is, you must first use the low power wide field of focus to locate the general area of action. Then you move up to higher power magnification to see the details of a particular area in the field. If you rush to the high power magnification first, you get confused as the images rush by too quickly. The harder you try to scan the field on high power magnification, the worse the result. Only by taking the binoculars away from your eyes, lining up your head with the general area of play, and then raising the binoculars to your eyes, can you get the play back into focus. Similarly, by reducing the magnification of the zoom lens, you see the total field. Then you locate the person you wish to photograph at higher power and zoom in at closer range.

Memory scanning at high power and close range is a reaction to stress. It produces words at too close range; words on the tip of your tongue, but out of focus of your consciousness. The best way to remember a word on the tip of your tongue is to go to lower magnification. First think of the category you are searching for — not the word itself. This scanning of the total field will help you localize the desired word in your field of memory. The exact word will then pop into your consciousness spontaneously.

Stress in the act of memory and recall can make you apply excessive coping efforts with poor results. Learning how to focus your efforts can make stress work for you rather than against you.

The STRESSCONTROL System emphasizes utilizing the painful stress symptoms as important sources of information. You must learn to decipher these symptoms and track them to their sources or root causes. This search for useful information contained within the stress symptom is called *focusing*. Having detected the source of the problem, the next task is finding a proper solution.

Most of us are quite good at solving our problems under calm circumstances. However, under stress and in pain, our coping mechanisms can falter or fail. We may become frantic prophets of gloom or we can become terrified and completely paralyzed by tension which builds each minute. Rather than using our intellect to find a solution, organized reasoning is stampeded into hasty action, panic, and confusion.

A key ingredient of the STRESSCONTROL System is positive psychological rehearsal of effective coping methods. We train people to plan positive courses of action to solve their stress problems and then to mentally rehearse these methods until they become second nature. This technique is patterned not after psychiatric principles but rather from my experiences as a pilot.

The value of positive rehearsal was brought home to me one night as I was about to take one of my final flying lessons before trying for my pilot's license. We were on a final approach to the runway and I was trying to stay one step ahead of events that, when you are landing an airplane, happen at 90 miles per hour.

The runway was lighted by a string of tiny lights which demarcated its borders. The pavement on which we were about to land was pitch black except for the beam of light coming from my airplane's landing light. Suddenly my instructor turned to me and said, "What would it be like to land with a malfunction of your landing lights?" "Terrible," I quickly replied. "Not as bad as it would be if it happened to you for the first time when your instructor wasn't around," he said, switching off the landing light. Trembling, I landed on a pitch black runway.

The next time it happened to me, I was a licensed pilot with no instructor around. When my landing light failed, the rehearsal he had given me in that simulated emergency made the subsequent one safely manageable. Flying instruction has taught me the life-saving benefits of positive rehearsal of coping methods. Each student pilot is put through simulated emergency situations again and again so that when real emergencies happen and the pilot is on his or her own, the stress of the situation will remain within constructive limits. The pilot learns to focus on the malfunction and rectify or compensate for it. Every good pilot on every flight mentally rehearses the possible emergencies that could occur in each stage of the flight and has a coping strategy available if it is needed. Good stress control in any situation requires an ability to focus on the problem and mentally *rehearse* positive solutions that can relieve the difficulties that may arise in a crisis situation.

Having identified the source of the stress through *focusing*, and armed by good stress control reflexes acquired through *positive rehearsal*, the individual must now *implement* these methods whenever a stressful situation is anticipated or when a symptom of stress is experienced. By using the STRESSCONTROL System, many people have learned to turn stress symptoms to their advantage. They use these body and mind signals as important barometers to gauge the pressures they are under and learn to set a winning pace through carefully regulating their stress levels.

If it is true that stress cannot be avoided, and is, in fact, necessary for productive life, then it must be controlled and optimized. Poorly controlled stress can be annoying, painful or even deadly. Stress that is handled properly can be an invigorating force in relationships, at work, and in self-development, providing one knows how to control its negative effects. Throughout this book we will review major life situations that cause stress; how it can get out of hand and work against you in personal and business relationships; at work, in sports, in childbirth, and in many other crucial domains — and how you can overcome the negative impact of stress.

1
Stress: I Can't Live without It

Are you aware of how your mind and body work? Probably not. In fact, none of us is even aware that aspects of our body and mind are in constant operation. Do you know for sure that your liver is working right now? How about your spleen, your adrenal glands, ovaries — I could go on and on. The point is that with the exception of heartbeats and breathing, nature has provided us with a very primitive, inadequate awareness about the operation of our body and its component parts.

Before birth, the embryo can feel and hear the beat of its own heart and its mother's as well. Throughout the years you are aware that your heart never stops beating — it is a miraculous pump that beats on the average of 70 times per minute for all the years of your life. When it skips even one beat, you become alarmed. There is no way to ignore a palpitation of the heart. You stop your activities and immediately tune in to your heartbeats to be sure that they are settling back to normal — and also to be sure that your heart is still beating. You sneak a reassuring feel of your pulse and then go back to what you were doing.

Nature has endowed us with acute survival instincts when it comes to the continued normal operation of the heart. Even the President of the United States will lay aside his most important duties if he begins to feel the squeezing chest pain of *angina pectoris*. This terrifying pain signals the person to relax and give the heart a rest. It may come on years before a heart attack, giving the person ample warning to change diet, lifestyle, have a bypass graft operation or take some other timely lifesaving measure.

The same goes for breathing. Even while you are asleep, if breathing is interrupted by an obstruction or is too shallow causing a lack of oxygen and excess carbon dioxide to accumulate in the body, you will sense it and wake up. Nature has provided us with good reflexes to cope with breathing problems.

With the exception of cardiac and respiratory functions, nature has shortchanged us as far as survival reflexes are concerned. Without sophisticated medical tests you don't know you have cancer often until it is too late to cure it. Your lungs can be half-rotted by tuberculosis and you will complain only of an "annoying cough." Leukemia, a killer, will hide for years behind "chronic fatigue." Nature's warning signals for most mental and physical catastrophes are, frankly, inadequate.

Perhaps the most important system in your body is the complex team of brain and hormonal activities which prepares your mind and body to deal with mental and physical challenges. Each time you face a situation that requires some ingenuity or extra effort to deal with it, your body, through an intricate reflex, mobilizes mental and physical energies smoothly and automatically. You look at your watch and see you are late for the train, so your heart begins to pound in preparation for running to catch it. Your boss says, "Get these proposals out by Friday!" Your mind becomes alert, awake and vigilant. Work pours from the tip of your ballpoint pen and you have trouble switching your brain off at night until you have delivered the finished proposals.

What is it that puts you into high gear so that you can get the job done efficiently and effectively? It's the body's and mind's *stress reaction*. We have a built-in alarm circuit system that activates these systems each time we face a challenge. Your mind is switched into the "on" position and becomes alert, awake and vigilant. Your body is activated by the same reflex: your heart begins to pump vigorously, your superficial blood vessels contract, blood is diverted away from the digestive tract to the muscles which have been drawn taut ready to spring into action. Termed the *fight or flight reaction,* it is nature's gift to the animal kingdom to ensure survival in emergency situations. When an animal is under attack, it must instantly be ready to run for its life or fight to the death. The animal becomes extremely alert and vigilant. Its muscles tense for a fight or life-saving escape through flight. Blood is diverted from the digestive tract where it is not needed, to the muscles where it is vitally required. The skin blood vessels clamp down in anticipation of possible injuries so that the animal will not bleed to death through a skin wound. Nature does a good job in the animal kingdom of wiring in sophisticated emergency survival systems — STRESS REACTIONS.

In the human species, this three-part reaction to danger — mental alertness, increased muscle activity and the spasm of superficial blood vessels can be extremely helpful. The soldier guarding the perimeter of his base at night needs to be alert, awake and vigilant. He must be aware of tiny intrusions that could spell danger. A crackle in the woods must instantly alert him. He must be vigilant and track down the source of that noise to eliminate the possibility of a hidden enemy, or to eliminate that enemy.

The soldier's physical reactions, like the animal's, anticipate possible sudden action and injury and provide survival reflexes to limit damage and maximize an effective physical response to the danger.

The mind's and body's stress reactions similarly prepare us to deal effectively with an infection, an operation, an argument with a taxi driver or any other challenge that we might encounter. Without the stress reaction we would get ill or die when confronted with any extraordinary demand since body and mind would be quickly overwhelmed. Stress helps us to raise our capacities to meet a challenge to survival. It is a life force that automatically goes into action to adjust body and mind systems to optimum coping levels — whether the challenge is meeting a work deadline, or surviving a heart transplant operation. But nature forgot one thing. While the "on" switch operates smoothly and automatically, the "off" switch frequently gets stuck. This can be a deadly flaw!

Nature's Greatest Triumph and Greatest Flaw — the Stress Thermostat

If you and I are not perfect, why do you assume Mother Nature is? The fact is that over millions of years of evolution, nature adjusts and improves a species for survival. In that sense, nature makes successive approximations toward perfection. In the interim, major deficits can exist in the human make-up. That is why we get sick and die. Nature leaves us unprepared or inadequately prepared for many environmental and social stresses, while over millions of years of evolution refining our bodies and minds to cope more effectively with our surroundings. "I can't wait that long!" you complain. "I won't be around in a million years. What can I do right now to compensate for these flaws in my creation?"

First of all, you can learn to be aware of these deficiencies and the impact they may have on your well-being. Then you can use your intelligence and available technology to compensate for these flaws. This principle is the foundation of modern medicine, surgery and psychiatry. And it is now being applied to the prevention of disease through stress control methods.

Let's go over the stress reaction once more and examine nature's goof. While we are endowed with a great emergency mechanism in the stress reaction, human crises last for days, months, sometimes years. The bank note coming due in six months that I may not be able to pay; my husband's constant traveling leaving me home alone to cope with the children and my loneliness simultaneously; a frustrating, low-paying job sandwiched in between two hours of commuting on jammed expressways.

Twentieth-century human challenges and crises continue for long periods or last indefinitely. Stress reactions are mobilized and remain in force for excessively long periods of time and eventually mutate into life-threatening forces from life-preserving forces. The mobilization of the heart and circulatory system over long crisis periods can lead to high blood pressure, strokes, heart attacks, migraine headaches, and heartbeat irregularities. The emergency diversion of blood from the intestinal tract to muscles can, over a long period, lead to indigestion and loss of appetite. Increases of muscle tension which are activated by crises, may be sustained as long as the crisis lasts: hours, days or more. Eventually, backache, tension headaches and muscle cramps will occur as the muscles become sore from silent over-exertion.

The overworked mind in a prolonged state of alertness, awakeness and vigilance produces anxiety, panic, feelings of dread and insomnia. Eventually, a nervous breakdown may occur when the taut mind is pressed beyond the point of coping with problems.

All body systems operate on a cybernetic principle — a feedback system akin to a thermostat. In the case of stress, this thermostat is triggered by environmental dangers as perceived by the individual. When a critical point is reached, the stress mechanism is thrown into action. There is an outpouring of stress hormones, a mobilization of the muscular and cardiovascular systems, and an alerting of the nervous system. This neurochemical reaction to stress is internally regulated by the body but it is not ordinarily under conscious control. Unfortunately, we are not aware of the level at which the thermostat is set! Only at the extreme do we realize that we are overworking our body and mind systems. On the verge of a nervous breakdown you frantically and most randomly reach for tranquilizers, TM, EST, psychotherapy, "anything that will work and help me get it together." High blood pressure has to be ready to blow out an artery in your brain before you realize that something ought to be done. Insomnia and indigestion remind you that you're much too tense. In other words, you've got to wait until after the problem occurs to know that you have a stress problem at all.

Society's progress has outstripped human evolution and adaptation when it comes to stress and so we have become a nation of pill takers, pot smokers and alcoholics. Valium outsells every other drug combined. Alcohol is abused by fully five percent of the nation's work force. And how many of your friends smoke grass because it is the only way they can relax? Our tensions, which arise from the way we live, cannot be eliminated. Car loans are here to stay. Marital problems and inflation won't go away. The aging process that frightens us in the midlife years cannot be avoided. They all cause stress reactions to be switched "on" and to stay "on." Nature hasn't yet endowed us with a natural awareness that the stress machinery in us has been switched to "on." We don't know at what level our stress thermostat is set except when it is past the red line, and none of us has a natural inborn ability to selectively shut down unnecessary components of the stress reaction.

"I'm going into a board meeting in five minutes. Let's see, I'll need 100 percent brain activation; thirty percent muscle activity (especially in my jaws, tongue and muscles of facial expression); and about fifteen percent power in the cardiovascular system. That should be sufficient." Possibly we'll operate that way in a million years. But today, the natural response is to go into the meeting and hope, "I won't get one of those damn migraines again." So with clenched jaw, drumming fingers, silently tensed scalp and back muscles and a heart that is running a 100-yard dash, we sit for two hours to the end of the meeting — burning up energy wastefully, producing unnecessary wear and tear on all body systems and operating always at less than optimum efficiency, given the nature of the crisis.

Nature's stress thermostat is dumb. It doesn't have the ability to discriminate between a street mugger and an unfavorable financial statement. And what's worse, we are mostly unaware that this misdirection of our stress reaction is going on until it's too late!

You Can Control Stress – The Marriage of Mind, Body and Transistor

By watching an infant learn to control and coordinate the movement of his hand, you will understand how you can learn to control stress. The infant constantly looks at his hand. He waves it, bangs it against the dangling mobile over the crib, watches it as it pushes a ball along and finally, through associating what he *sees* with what he *feels* in the muscles and joints of the arm and hand, he learns to operate the hand smoothly without having to look at it. It is a principle of human biology that if you can be sharply aware of a function, you can learn to control that function. The infant uses *visual feedback* to sharpen and coordinate muscular activity in the hand and eventually the hand is precisely programmed to operate effectively without visual feedback. This principle is being widely applied to teaching tennis and skiing. Videotape replays of your style give you visual information that helps you refine the muscular coordination required for top tennis or skiing performance. Dancers have long practiced in front of mirrors before performing in front of audiences for that reason.

The reason you cannot control your stress is that you cannot *see* the stress thermostat and thus you cannot learn how to regulate it voluntarily. As you sit here reading this book, you have no reliable awareness of your level of muscle or cardiovascular activity. As long as your muscles are not hurting, you don't know if they are set at a level of tension a scant distance from a cramp or pain or at a relaxed level. You cannot perceive your own blood pressure or level of blood vessel contraction. Only when your hands feel too cold are you aware of a stress reaction in your blood vessels. Not knowing how to *tune in* to these functions, you cannot focus your mind on them and practice voluntary control over them.

With the advent of space age electronics, a major breakthrough occurred in the field of stress control and preventive medicine. Electronic devices were produced at reasonable cost which could pick up minute signals from the brain and muscles and convert these to sound and visual information. These devices could be used as electronic mirrors to reflect specific stress reactions, providing immediate visual and auditory information to an individual connected to the equipment. Suddenly, medical science has at its disposal a set of "eyes" and "ears" that can see and hear the stress thermostat in a highly accurate way. It became apparent, when people were attached to these machines, they could quickly learn to control their own stress thermostats. The *feedback* of information telling the individual at what level the muscle tension thermostat was set quickly allowed that person to learn to reset it at a much lower level. The same learning occurred when skin temperature information was fed back to a person. Within minutes, the individual could learn to relax blood vessels in the hand and raise skin temperature by many degrees.

The medical applications came quickly. Individuals trained on these machines could learn to prevent migraine and tension headaches; cure the early phases of high blood pressure; be relieved of anxiety and insomnia; and even reduce to a minimum severe pain associated with cancer and other deadly diseases. Biofeedback began to be talked about and used, even feared, as some individuals wondered whether we would become a nation of robots — transistorized, bionic men and women. Nevertheless, stress control programs, assisted by biofeedback equipment, have demonstrated increasing usefulness and along with that have gained wider and wider public acceptance.

The keys to the control of stress are:

1. The ability to **focus** on the function
2. The **rehearsal** of stress-alleviating methods
3. **Application** of these methods in the face of situations which unnecessarily mobilize stress reactions

People who have learned biofeedback relaxation methods can quickly dispense with the use of the electronic device, just as it isn't necessary to be videotaped forever in order to maintain a synchronized tennis serve. Once learned, the body and mind are reprogrammed and do not require the *feedback* over an extended time.

The marriage of mind, body and transistor has allowed us to correct nature's oversight and let us directly control our stress thermostat.

The Chief Misconception about Stress is that It Is Synonymous with Aggravation or an Overload of Hardships

When we think about what causes stress, our mind conjures up an image out of our experience that is usually negative or painful:

> I couldn't sleep last night. My husband was on the road for two weeks and I was wondering what he did last night. He sounded so cold and distant on the phone — almost guilty. Does he have a girlfriend in Philadelphia? I really get upset thinking about this.

*The doctor is still in the operating room with your mother —
the operation is taking a little longer than we expected.*

*This is Captain Renfrew speaking. We've had a small mal-
function in our landing gear and will be heading back to La
Guardia to get it repaired.*

*Mommy — daddy. Why are you getting divorced? Why can't
I live with both of you?*

We have a notion stress is activated only by human suffering
and when we keep clear of traumatic situations we elude stress as
well. This is not so! Consider a situation in which I found myself
only a few weeks ago.

I was invited to attend a black-tie party given to support a local
charity. The host, a famous New York plastic surgeon, held the
affair in his palatial Manhattan townhouse. My wife and I were
standing together exchanging the usual cocktail party niceties
with another couple. Suddenly, the three-man band played a fan-
fare and the tinkle of glasses and chatter subsided. The host announced, "We have a treat in store for you — a fashion show." At
once, a spotlight was switched on and focused on the top of the
spiral staircase. My wife knows me to be a self-confessed admirer
of redheads, so when a luscious readhead stepped into the spotlight, my heart quickened and my wife's grip on my arm reminded
me that she knew what I was thinking. To a bouncy tune, the
redhead descended the staircase as the host announced, "Furs and
lady's undergarments by Oscar Pierre of Paris!" As the redhead
reached our level, the fur slid off her body revealing a flimsy
negligee clinging and swaying around an exquisite body.

The redhead started toward us. My wife's grip tightened and my
hands were ice. She approached to within inches of my body and
then slid by me in three sections pelvis, chest, red lips. *That was
stress* — and I loved every minute of it!

Stress of major proportions can be caused by desired events — a
promotion, getting married, or buying your dream house. This
brings us to the central issue concerning the causation of stress.
All circumstances which produce change also produce stress.

Stress is activated within us as a means of coping with and adapting to change, either *good* or *bad*. Since change is an ever-present aspect of life, there is no escape from stress. Stress must either be controlled and used to best advantage, or it will wear you down, due to the primitive tendency we all have to "call out the troops," no matter what the nature of the stress.

Here is a checklist of one year's life events that involve significant amounts of stress. It has been determined by Drs. Thomas H. Holmes and Richard H. Rahe* that if you score above 150 accumulated points, you are subject to high levels of stress sometimes associated with emotional and/or physical illness.

Life Event	Mean Value
1. Death of spouse	100
2. Divorce	73
3. Marital separation	65
4. Jail term	63
5. Death of close family member	63
6. Personal injury or illness	53
7. Marriage	50
8. Fired at work	47
9. Marital reconciliation	45
10. Retirement	45
11. Change in health of family member	44
12. Pregnancy	40
13. Sexual difficulties	39
14. Gain of new family member	39
15. Business readjustment	39
16. Change in financial state	38
17. Death of close friend	37
18. Change to different line of work	36
19. Change in number of arguments with spouse	35
20. Mortgage over $10,000	31
21. Foreclosure of mortgage or loan	30
22. Change in responsibilities at work	29
23. Son or daughter leaving home	29

*See Holmes, T.H. and Rahe, R.H.: "The Social Readjustment Rating Scale," JOURNAL OF PSYCHOSOMATIC RESEARCH Vol. II (1967), pp. 213–218.

24.	Trouble with in-laws	29
25.	Outstanding personal achievement	28
26.	Spouse begins or stops work	26
27.	Beginning or ending school	26
28.	Change in living conditions	25
29.	Revision of personal habits	24
30.	Trouble with boss	23
31.	Change in work hours or conditions	20
32.	Change in residence	20
33.	Change in schools	20
34.	Change in recreation	19
35.	Change in church activities	19
36.	Change in social activities	18
37.	Mortgage or loan less than $10,000	17
38.	Change in sleeping habits	16
39.	Change in number of family get-togethers	15
40.	Change in eating habits	15
41.	Vacation	13
42.	Christmas	12
43.	Minor violations of the law	11

Before you panic, feeling doomed to illness by your stress score, remember that the results are statistical — not all people will break down; just a higher percentage than average. Also, you aren't helpless. You are going to learn to cope with stress and change.

Coping with Stress

In your efforts to cope with stress there are three domains of major concern:

1. Stressful Life Events
2. The Way You Cope with Them
— The Stress Control Approach

3. Your Personality Structure — The Psychotherapeutic Approach

Traditionally, an individual suffering the ravages of stress would eventually end up at a psychiatrist's or psychologist's office looking for relief. If psychotherapy was recommended, it would have as its goal the rebuilding of the individual's personality to remove internal conflicts and self-defeating neurotic patterns. The goal of psychotherapy is to rebuild you inside so that you can learn to face the stresses of life more effectively. The stress control approach is to study and reeducate your coping mechanisms. When you are reprogrammed to cope with stress more effectively on a mental and physical level, your life experiences will be more productive and enjoyable. While inner conflicts arising from childhood are not exposed and explained, the *effects* of poor learning in early life *can* be changed. Better coping mechanisms *can* be learned directly — without reference to your entire early life history. The approach of the psychotherapist and the approach of a stress control program are complementary. Choose one or the other and you benefit. Choose both and you profit enormously.

Let's consider the two levels of importance in a stress control program: your coping mechanisms and stressful life events.

You can construct a vital stress control formula out of these concepts that can guide you in your day-to-day dealings with stress:

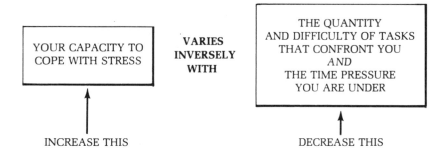

You can increase your capacity to cope with stress three ways:

1. **Reduce** the quantity and/or difficulty of the tasks that confront you.
2. **Reduce** the time pressure you are under to complete the tasks.
3. **Increase** your coping skills through reeducation.

Let's apply this to a marital crisis. Your husband announces to you that he has been unhappy with the relationship for a long time and lately has been considering a divorce. You also have grown weary of the unending series of gripes and battles. Both of you would like to save the marriage but don't know an effective strategy to implement. "Maybe we ought to buy that country house and new car that we have been denying ourselves. Perhaps if we got into more things together, we'd begin to loosen up and feel better." *Wrong!*

Many couples in a marital crisis go on a buying and new activity spree. They try to fill a void in their lives by a frenzy of new purchases or new activities. Rather than improving their ability to cope with the marital crisis, it often undermines it. Referring to the formula, the couple would do better to *reduce* the quantity and difficulty of tasks confronting them. They might dedicate themselves to learning to enjoy just one evening a week together. "Let's start dating again. We'll decompress our relationship and make no demands on each other six days out of seven. We'll just go our separate ways without guilt or obligation. Let's learn how to enjoy only Saturday together. We'll hang loose all week and then really try to be fresh and eager to enjoy our one day together. If that goes well — we'll try a whole weekend together and build from there."

"Why don't you give me your decision?" another woman demanded of her husband. "Either you want me or you don't. Stop procrastinating. I can't stand the uncertainty."

"But I just don't know," her husband replied. "I'm confused. There are so many good things about the marriage I don't want to lose and yet so many problems with it — I just can't cope with it or decide to end it at this point."

"If you don't, *I will*. I can't live this way," the wife insisted.

This is a familiar scene that precedes the demise of many a salvageable relationship. Increasing the time pressure for coping decreases the person's ability to cope with crisis. Why do it to yourself if it is unnecessary?

Lastly, marital therapy can reeducate and upgrade a couple's coping skills for making an intimate relationship more successful. The stress control formula for managing a marital crisis is:

1. **Reduce** the quantity and difficulty of the tasks confronting the couple. Do LESS; enjoy it MORE.
2. **Reduce** the time pressure for solving the problem.
3. **Increase** coping skills through marital counseling.

Later in this book (Chapter 7) we describe in detail seven key areas for reducing stress in marital life through improving coping skills.

Whenever someone puts me on the spot and increases time pressure on me for a decision, I respond, "Would you like a *slow* YES or a *fast* NO?" That usually cools things off.

If someone tries to influence me to take on more tasks than I can handle, I usually respond, "A *small* YES is better than a *big* NO." They usually get the message and scale down their demands to where I'm likely to accept their request.

The Stress-Intensifying Personality

Some personality types seem to be designed to magnify stresses rather than to cope with and master challenges. These *stress-intensifying* personalities are poison either to have or be with because their effects are contagious.

1. The Type A personality* not only puts him or herself under time pressures but tries to impose it on you too. Type A's can't do enough in one time frame. They are never

*Friedman, M. and Rosenmann, R.H., Type A Behavior and Your Heart, (New York: Alfred A. Knopf, 1974).

satisfied with what you do either. The Type A personality has
an overdose of internal aggression which constantly spills
over into other people's lives. "I don't get ulcers — I give
them!" said one Type A business executive while being
examined for epigastric pain. He was right. Instead, his pain
was finally diagnosed as a heart attack and he almost died in
the coronary care unit.

2. *The Worrier* sees pain and problems as ubiquitous or in
hot pursuit of him. He identifies no personal internal strength
or ability to cope — even though it is present. His mind never
rehearses positive solutions — only disaster scenarios. Life is
designed around running and hiding from fears rather than
satisfying needs. If you try to help, he is only too happy to
revere your strength and contrast it to his own weakness, thus
intensifying his feelings of helplessness and dependency on
you.

3. *The Guilt-Ridden* is governed by an internal tyrannical
conscience. While he is able to recognize he does have some
internal personal strength, when he starts to cope with a
problem he feels guilty about how long it's taking, the
discomfort it might be causing other people, whether the
solution will meet with other people's approval. The
guilt-ridden person adds an overdose of conscience to an
already difficult life task and is shot down by the double
barrels of external life and internal strife.

4. *The Perfectionist* is pervaded with such intense and
unrealistic optimism about himself and others that the end
result is always a feeling of failure. "You can do it better," his
personality endlessly insists, causing him to judge himself
and others always short of their full potential. "More tasks
can always be handled — and they can be handled better and
faster," his mind coaxes and cajoles. The Perfectionist
eventually overdoses on optimism and fails to function due to
his self-imposed ideals that can never be met and the feelings
of failure and disappointment thus engendered.

5. *The Prove-I'm Right-At-Any-Cost Person* is a vindication
addict. He can't settle for the conclusion, "You can't win
them all." In fact, if you convincingly prove him wrong, it

only whets his appetite for more vindication and makes him struggle with you all the harder to prove he is right — no matter what the cost in bad feelings, time wasted, logic and twisted facts, and the stress imposed on both of you. If you feed his addiction for vindication by agreeing with him, don't be surprised if he takes the opposite side of the issue and renews the argument. He thrives on vindication and without feeling criticized or opposed he cannot fight to uphold his convictions. Many such people enter law or politics where there is an infinite reservoir of opportunities to feed their addiction.

Stay away from these people and you will avoid much unnecessary stress. If you are one of them, then I suggest you begin searching for a good psychiatrist or psychologist. It might be the wisest investment you ever made and the most humane and generous thing you can do for those around you.

2
Stress and Your Mind

Recollections of My Own Psychoanalysis

A dozen years ago I decided to do something about my own mental distress. I was nearing the midway point in my psychiatric training and had had enough experience with disturbed patients to begin to understand the source of my own mental suffering. I decided to enter psychoanalysis as the way to learn techniques for coping with my own problems.

Dr. Pinard's receptionist directed me to sit in his waiting room until he finished with a patient. Glancing nervously around the waiting room I searched for clues to Pinard's personality in order to prepare me for the interview with him which I desired but feared. "He likes Impressionistic art," I remarked to myself. "No news magazines on his rack, only timeless publications like *Architecture in America* and *Art News*. There's nothing in this waiting room to connect me with the troubles of the world."

"Dr. Lecker, I'm Dr. Pinard. Please follow me." I was startled by his sudden presence and followed him to his consulting room with growing panic. "How will I start — what will I say — I'll look like a fool — maybe he'll think I'm a psychotic." I worked myself over as I trailed him into his dimly lit consulting room and sat in the chair he designated.

"Well, Dr. Lecker, tell me how I can help you," he began. I gulped, hesitated, wished I had never decided to start this process, then gathered my nerve and explained.

"Dr. Pinard, you're probably going to think me foolish or my problems trivial but, well, I really think I'm *too sane*. And it's boring me to death. I need a reason for everything I do — I can't act foolishly or spontaneously just for the hell of it. I'm a wet blanket in a crowd because I'm intractably serious and reasonable while my friends are all irrational, fun-loving, and sometimes juvenile. I envy them — they tolerate me. This unremitting sanity, of which I am a victim, affects everything I do. Even when I read *Playboy,* my eyes are drawn more to the copy than to the nudes as if I must understand the rationale behind the presentation of each picture. So I end up reading that 'Cindy Flame from Portland has always admired firemen,' thus purporting to explain why she ended up pictured in the nude caressing a firehose in the June issue. There's no question in my mind, Dr. Pinard, that I'm afflicted with some form of malignant sanity that's draining and choking all the joy out of my life. Can you help me? Can you make me, I hate to say it, crazier than I am. Without overdoing it!" I hastened to add.

Pinard puffed twice on his pipe and slowly turned to the credenza behind him. He picked up a small silver tray in one hand and reached into one of two pewter urns behind him, retrieving something which he placed on the tray. He turned back in my direction and extended the tray to me. "Take it," he said, as I glanced down. I was startled to discover a fortune cookie reposing on the tray. "Food for the body and food for the soul," Pinard said, solemnly urging me to take the cookie.

Breaking it open, I pulled out a sliver of paper on which was written, "Wider horizons await you." I was filled with anticipation and asked, "Does this mean you can help me?" Pinard puffed again on his pipe and nodded in the direction of his couch. I walked over and lay down, reassured that Pinard would help me out of the sterile emotional maze I was in and that I would, through this process, learn to be more carefree, more spontaneous, childlike when I felt like it, able to look a nude straight in the bust, and willing to sacrifice reason for happiness when I wanted to. He would help me to be crazier than I had been for years and yet less crazy than I feared I would be if my sterile life continued.

I saw Pinard three years in all. The same pattern more-or-less occurred at each session. I complained about everything that had occurred in my life since childhood or since the last therapy session. He extended the silver tray to me with its fortune cookie on it. I broke open the cookie (an annoying thing to do when you are lying down because you get crumbs inside your shirt) and I dutifully read the sliver of paper with interest (at the beginning) but became increasingly annoyed as the months went by.

Finally I complained angrily, "Pinard, this is not working! So I've gotten a lot of things off my chest in the past few months and am overloaded with fortune cookie wisdom. But I don't feel better — and that's what I came here for in the first place, isn't that right?"

"Wrong," Pinard coolly answered.

"What do you mean?" I replied, pained and puzzled.

Pinard went on, "You didn't come to feel better in this office. You wanted to feel better in the context of your life. When you first stated your complaint to me about being too sane, you were on the right track. You had set your own goal for therapy and you did something to implement that goal — you found a psychoanalyst and engaged in a process or interaction with me. Since you've been in therapy, you've complained about a lot of frustrations and unmet needs. These, too, are goals that need to be achieved. What have you done to implement solutions to these problems?"

I hesitated just short of almost saying, "I come here every week and read what is in the fortune cookie . . ." and then the wisdom of his remarks penetrated my mind. I had always been a "thinker" rather than a "doer," I realized. I figure out quite easily what my frustrations and complaints are but then I cherish the problems rather than the solutions. No matter how many fortune cookies of wisdom he hands me, I'll never get better until I change my own style from thinking to doing.

I shifted gears in therapy, placing more emphasis in my sessions on mentally and emotionally rehearsing solutions to my problems rather than on simply making Pinard into my emotional garbage collector. As I found out quickly, this produced a bonanza of results. I would *focus* on a problem in my life and then *rehearse* a solution to it with Pinard sitting behind me, ready to remind me that I *did* have the resources to implement it, despite my early experiences which had programmed my mind to believe that my parents or their surrogates (like my boss, or Pinard himself) were responsible for rescuing me. I learned to take more charge of my own life and to *act*, even when I was uncertain of the outcome of that action. "I'll be O.K., no matter how it turns out. I'll handle the consequences," I learned to say to myself and believe. It worked! I got crazier and happier. Finally, I decided that I was crazy enough and didn't need any more therapy. Pinard agreed and we ended our relationship.

Focusing on the problem. That's a fine thing to do. But many therapies neglect the process of *coping*. Learning how to get out and *do* something that will change your life for the better must not be omitted from therapeutic or self-help approaches that deal with the stresses of life. As in my, only partly facetious, autobiographical vignette, therapy can become a cop-out for life, feeding you the opportunity for endless reflection in your therapist's office (as long as your money holds out). Instead, therapy, or the process of reflection it is supposed to engender, must become a springboard for *action*. It is a preparation for coping, as well as an opportunity to assess the results of your coping efforts. If you participate in a therapy that doesn't lead to more effective action on your part *outside of therapy*, then your efforts and money are being wasted. Use therapy as a temporary mental refuge, allowing you to safely think, feel and mentally rehearse any and all responses to your life dilemmas. Then go out into the world and *do it!*

The Psychiatrist as Guru and Used Car Salesman

Having been a practicing psychiatrist for ten years, I'm convinced that psychiatrists and psychologists are the best salespeople in the history of civilization. We have the most difficult product in the world to sell and the most customer resistance to overcome. You see, we have to sell you on *you!* Or more precisely, we have to help you to decide to once again use aspects of your mind and personality that you have discarded as troublesome or useless.

Medical doctors have it easy by comparison. You break a leg. They say, "I'll fix it up like new." You trust them, knowing by experience that you have always had two sound legs and, even though one is broken, you can rely on the fact that it will soon be in as good shape as the healthy one. As a customer, you have had a good experience with the product — your leg — so you expect good results from the treatment.

Psychiatrists and psychologists have a far more difficult product to sell. "I want you to loosen up and start feeling your emotions again," we say.

"Oh yeah, I've had only trouble from those goddamned emotions for years. Thanks but no thanks," you reply.

"Let's work on your communication with each other," we say to a distressed couple heading for divorce. "After fifteen years of him beating my brains out emotionally, I'm not sure I can or want to communicate with my husband any more."

As a salesman, I'd rather sell you Fratter-Snappers than mental health. If you said, "I don't need any Fratter-Snappers," I could reply, "Why? Have you ever tried any? How do you know they won't help you enjoy life more until you have tried them?" At least I could play on your naiveté as a customer to convince you to try something *new* — and I could throw in a few testimonials about how your neighbors' lives have improved through the use of Fratter-Snappers.

But when it comes to selling you on reviving aspects of your mind and emotions that you have buried, I am at a disadvantage as a salesman because the *product is used* and your previous experience with it has been largely *unsatisfactory*. What a shame, because when it comes to dealing with stresses that affect your mind, you can't afford to operate on two cylinders. You need access to all your mental and emotional resources in order to cope with life. Where there is a hidden or discarded emotion or ability, it has to be uncovered, revamped, and put into full use again. You need all the help you can get in dealing with stress and your chief resource is yourself — your mind, your emotions, and your body.

The Dynamic Stability of the Mind and Forces That Upset the Applecart

I don't hesitate to criticize Mother Nature for the shortcomings with which she has endowed us. But I must give credit where credit is due. The mind is an utterly amazing creation — all six billion cells of it. Unlike the body's primitive self-destructive reaction to stress, the mind has a built-in mechanism of self-preservation. One of its most unusual and least known properties is its *dynamic stability* — its ability to set itself right after being disturbed (as long as you don't meddle in the process).

Do you remember the punch toy you had as a child? It stood upright and had a sand-filled base. If you hit it, it swayed and then returned to the upright position. You could knock it over until it hit the ground horizontally and then it would pop erect immediately. The only way you could get it to lie flat was to *hold* it down. That property of self-correction is called *dynamic stability*.

When I first learned to fly an airplane I was introduced to the property of dynamic stability once again. Every airplane is built to fly straight and level. If you push the nose over into a dive, the plane builds up speed — the wings develop more lifting power at the higher speed — and the plane tends to level off. Point the nose to the sky and the plane slows down — the wings lose lift at the lower speed — and the plane will level off again. If you want the plane to nose dive into the ground, you have to point the nose earthward and force the wheel (or stick) to remain forward, overcoming the plane's natural tendency to come spontaneously out of a deadly dive. Keep your hands off, and the inherent design of the plane will tend to solve the problem itself.

The human mind is also designed with a property of dynamic stability. Subject it to stress and it bends, but doesn't break; and then it springs back to normal as long as you keep HANDS OFF. In terms of the human mind this bending process under stress takes place as a natural tendency of the mind to regress, relax and unload tensions. Subjected to overwhelming stress, we get to a point where we say, "I quit; I can't take it anymore. I need a vacation or I need help — I can't cope." We yell, cry, rage irrationally, are afraid, become infantile and dependent temporarily — and then it's all over. The stress has passed, we feel under less pressure; time and regression have given us the respite we needed to gather our energies and we resume our adult posture once more, ready to cope actively with the disturbing forces in our lives.

Many of us can't leave well enough alone. We don't allow the dynamic stability of our minds to rescue us. We fight the controls like an unskilled pilot risking death by not trusting in the inherently good design of his aircraft. We say, "I can't quit — even temporarily. I can take it."

"I won't show my emotions — that is a weakness."

"Who needs help — if I ask for help, they'll think I'm not capable anymore. They'll lose faith in me." We fight the lifesaving regression that allows the mind to bend under pressure; and then suddenly the mind *snaps*. Mental regression then becomes irresistible and may become irreversible as well. "Poor Charlie — he never was sick a day in his life. He worked like a horse and never complained — carried his load all alone. Then he had this nervous breakdown. I can't understand it. Poor guy, he never could get that old zip and energy back."

Charlie fought against his own natural dynamic stability and lost. Many people do the same with inevitably similar results. Some permit themselves to regress and recover only when it is camouflaged in a socially acceptable way. They need alcohol or marijuana to justify the release of emotions. They accept help surreptitiously from a close confidant, doctor, or clergyman but never seek it openly in their work setting where it is most needed. They deal with their own fears of dependency by becoming overpowering and controlling with their subordinates at work, or with their children or even with their spouses.

Mental stress is present when you feel the temptation to regress, to quit, to give up. But, if you are one of those who fights against your own dynamic stability, you will know you are under mental stress when you feel an irresistible pressure to prove your competence, your control, and your independence. Failure to recognize the presence of mental stress gives it the jump on you. You can't afford that — no matter how strong and competent you fancy yourself.

The successful treatment of a nervous breakdown always involves the three key elements of a stress control formula:

1. *Reduce* the quantity and complexity of tasks that confront you (through hospitalization, a leave of absence from work, or even a few days of vacation).
2. *Reduce* the time pressure on you for dealing with stress. If you can't do this spontaneously, tranquilizers (when prescribed by a psychiatrist), or meditation will slow you down and reduce your anxiety about getting things done immediately.
3. *Increase* coping skills through psychotherapy and education about the causes of your stress and ways to cope.

A good stress control plan directs you to take the pressure off temporarily and let your mind revive its energies. Only then will its own dynamic stability help you to bounce back to full capacity. An even better idea is, of course, to recognize mental stress by its earliest manifestations and learn to lower the pressures on yourself through temporary regression — even if you only take an hour or an afternoon off to play and relax so that the inherent dynamic stability of your mind can restore normal functioning quickly and effectively.

The Mind as a Tool for Satisfying Needs

One of the chief ways we differ from other species in the animal kingdom is the way in which we use our mind to satisfy our needs. In the animal, needs are satisfied through instinct. Hunger or lust, when felt by the animal, set in motion an almost automatic behavioral sequence: foraging for food, directed by a keen sense of smell; ritualistic courting ending inevitably in copulation.

How different for the human with a hunger for food and sex. "Better not eat too much or I'll get fat and be unattractive. I'll have to get a better job so that I can earn more money, buy better-looking clothes, be able to frequent better places, pick up more desirable women, and with a lot of practice, I'll learn how to get across to a girl, maybe even to have sex with her or get serious with her or something . . ." The human has fractured instinctual behavior: a strong and definite beginning; a no-man's land in between; and a definite end in mind. The in between activity is what makes us so much more intelligent than every other species. The *lack of automaticity* of our instincts gets us started, but leaves us dangling in midair, hungering for food or panting for sexual satisfaction. We then have to figure out how to satisfy our needs. This pressures us to explore, invent, innovate and create intricate and prolonged solutions for our needs. That is what develops the latent potential of our mind. Put an infant in a crib and feed it, protect it and never frustrate or stimulate it and the resulting adult will be dull at the least or severely retarded at the worst.

Nature has endowed us with the ability to *want*, but no automatic instincts to satisfy these requirements. Instead, we are endowed with superior doing and judging abilities and left on our own to figure out solutions for satisfying our needs. We must develop our mind power in order to reduce the pressure from our instincts. The most important and vulnerable aspects of our minds reside in how we coordinate our abilities *to want, to do* and *to judge.*

WANTING AND ITS STRESS POINTS

We are all familiar with our basic wants: food, shelter, companionship, sex and security are some major ones built-in at birth. A peculiar thing can occur when one of these basic needs is consistently denied or if we are traumatized in the process of satisfying a need. We substitute another need in its place and satisfy that need for which there is a more accessible satisfaction. Hence, the person who finds it hard to gain social acceptance and satisfaction may resort to overeating. The person with an insecurity over sexual prowess substitutes for this requirement a magnificent shelter — Georgian columns, concrete swimming pool and all. The problem with oversatisfying these substitute needs is that the basic need still presses silently for satisfaction. Having learned to misinterpret its signal, we invest even more energy in the false solution, leaving fewer resources to deal with the important but hidden vital need.

Consider the case of a successful physician I treated whose father died when he was a child. He was raised by a competent and loving mother but always had great insecurity about his masculinity. He turned to his profession and became an extremely competent physician — proving himself in an arena where he could easily measure his success in terms of professional status, numbers of patients in his practice and money earned. When he began to have marital and sexual difficulties, he threw himself even more vigorously into his practice and retreated from the problems of his home life. The marriage a shambles, his wife finally sued for divorce, forcing him to recognize the failure of their relationship.

He spent the first several months in therapy with me sparring intellectually in an effort to demonstrate his professional prowess. He was good, even excellent, at understanding the technical and theoretical problems of his marriage. However, he was lousy at living in it. Finally I told him, "The only way you are going to win is to lose." He was puzzled and disturbed. I went on. "As long as you insist on being the competent doctor in control of the situation here, you will never get to the core of the problem and its solution. But if you agree to give up on being competent as a doctor in this setting, you may learn to recognize the lonely and frightened little boy in you that lost his father in childhood. If you can tune in to that part of yourself, I'm sure we can help your wife to recognize that aspect of you as well. She can learn to be loving, encouraging and supportive when you feel most insecure. If you want to *win* as a man and as a husband, you must teach yourself when to *lose* as far as being the intellectual master of all situations is concerned." He did learn eventually that it was appropriate to lose sometimes and in the process, he gained back his marriage and his sexual confidence without diminishing his stature as a physician one bit.

Some wants are programmed into us by experience. They are not basic or essential to life. They may even be overtly destructive, but they become as firmly entrenched in us as our real and vital needs through mental association:

I smoke because it helps me get through stressful situations.

Why do I drink? Look, the boys always get together after work for a few belts and some laughs.

If I don't take a Valium, I can't get on a plane.

I know I put up with her insults and criticisms in front of our guests and relatives. Listen, she's a good woman at heart. She keeps a good house, looks after the kids . . . .

These programmed-in needs are mentally but not *actually* connected with vital needs:

- Cigarette smoking *doesn't* help increase your capacity to cope with stressful situations.
- Drinking *isn't* essential to intimate socializing with friends.
- Valium *doesn't* keep the airplane airborne.
- Insults from your wife *aren't* essential to her skills as a mother and housekeeper.

If you want to function more effectively with respect to your needs and wants, you may wish to complete a table like this for each strong need you feel. Then add up the score and see if it's worth your while to continue the same need-satisfying behavior. Consider, as an example, this table on heavy social drinking:

THE EFFECTS OF MY NEED-SATISFYING BEHAVIOR

	1 Reduces Stress	4 Intensifies Stress
Helps Me Emotionally/Physically		
Hurts Me Emotionally/Physically	✓	✓
Brings Me Closer to People		✓
Causes Rifts Between Me and People		✓
Makes Me Proud of Myself		
Makes Me Ashamed and Guilty		✓
Hurts Others Who Are Important to Me		✓
Satisfies and Protects Others Who Are Important To Me		
TOTAL		

WHAT MY NEEDS ARE	THE THINGS I DO TO SATISFY MY NEEDS
1. Socializing	Need No. 1 a. Get together with friends after work
2.	b. Drink alcohol
3.	c. Tell stories
4.	d. Watch sports on T.V.
5.	
6.	etc. . . .
etc. . . .	

DOING — AND ITS STRESS POINTS

What happens when you finally decide to do something to improve your life? Why do some people find the process of self-improvement so painful and threatening? Transitions of any sort are stressful. While people may intensely dislike the life they are currently leading, in order to change they must relinquish the familiar — the status quo — and begin a search for something better. Casting about for a better way to live means you must accept and even welcome a prolonged period of uncertainty. It is that transitional period of instability that people fear and often avoid, leading to either a retreat from self-improvement or an impulsive solution in an attempt to shorten the period of instability. Changing requires that you undo aspects of your life, search for better solutions, and then know when enough change has occurred.

The sequence is:

1. UNDOING THE PRESENT SITUATION
2. INSTABILITY AND CHANGE
3. KNOWING WHEN TO STOP

You must be able to:

- Define what it is that you want to undo — *focus* on the critical block to your ability to cope with life.
- Mentally *rehearse* positive solutions to the problem.
- *Initiate* change at an appropriate time.
- Learn to *tolerate and even welcome the anxiety* associated with the instability and change.
- Learn to *set goals* in advance so that you won't get stuck in a process of change-for-the-sake-of-change and overshoot your mark.

Stress points of this process are:

- Not being able to *focus* on what is essential to change and, therefore, taking a shotgun approach, setting too many changes in motion at once, far more than you can handle.

- Getting stuck in a mental rut of rehearsing your fears of disaster and failure rather than contemplating positive ways of guiding yourself through the period of instability effectively.
- Failing to time the onset of change properly so that you don't have enough time, energy or resources to carry it through
- When going through the period of instability that necessarily accompanies change, panicking and making rash moves to cope with the tension — or putting a premature halt to the process, short of your objectives.
- Having fuzzy goals so that you're never quite sure when and how much to do — you never know when you have reached your goal.

Recently I treated a woman who was an Olympic gold medal class masochist. Her husband, his relatives, and even her own children, including one preschooler, took advantage of her and abused her in public. She suffered in silence for years and finally, even though her mind still came back for more, her stomach gave out. She developed a severe gastric ulcer which finally resulted in the surgical removal of most of her stomach. When she still suffered "ulcer" pains after surgery, her surgeon insisted she see a psychiatrist since neither ulcer nor stomach were in her body any longer.

In short order, we were able to establish that her continuing pain was a psychosomatic phenomenon, a body expression of pain originating in her punishing relationships with everyone in her life. Through the course of some months of therapy, she agreed to make changes in her relationships with people. She vowed to insist that people show her consideration and respect as a condition of her remaining in a relationship with them.

Things went well with her children. She put her foot down and they responded quickly and positively, relieved they could finally respect their own mother. Her husband and in-laws presented a stickier problem. She decided to press for change with them just after her husband had been laid off from work. She insisted on better treatment and more respect. Her husband, caught up in his own disappointment, rebelled and left the home for a temporary separation, aided and abetted by his "understanding family." Realizing that her timing was poor in launching a major campaign to revamp her marriage, she relented, apologized to him for her insensitivity and they reunited.

When he was securely back in his job, she again attempted to shift the equilibrium of their relationship toward more justice and understanding for herself. Her husband again rebelled, not leaving home this time, but engaging in vicious verbal attacks on her which in the past had intimidated her into silent acceptance of his punishment and neglect. While not at all accustomed to assert herself, she held her ground with my encouragement and gave him an ultimatum. "We go into marital therapy together or you leave this house and family. I don't want to be an emotional sparring partner for your frustrations, and you don't need a wife whom you can't respect or admire." She gritted her teeth as he packed his bags threatening to leave for good — but she didn't waver. "If I have to survive as a single parent, I will — many other women do and I will, too." He turned from his suitcase and said, "This is the first time in years that I have felt respect for you. What's your psychiatrist's phone number — I want to make an appointment to see him."

She set her goals (undoing her poor relationships).

She stuck by her guns through a period of turmoil.

And she stopped the process of change when her relationships with her family had improved, resisting the temptation to "overshoot" and pay them back for the years of suffering they had inflicted on her, which would only have reignited destructive hostility in her life.

JUDGING — AND ITS STRESS POINTS

After we know which wants are most important to us, and we establish what we can do to satisfy these needs, we judge ourselves as to our manner and success in attaining our goals. Sometimes we are reasonable with ourselves. At times we are excessively harsh or lax. Some of us tend to the extremes too consistently.

An attorney whom I was treating set such impossible goals for himself that he suffered stress-related symptoms of two varieties. He had recurrent and severe migraine headaches, and he pushed himself so hard at work, always fearing failure, that he began to lose efficiency and effectiveness in his work due to sheer fatigue. His partners considered him to be a first-rate trial lawyer. His record of acquittals for his clients was nothing short of spectacular. Despite this, he pushed himself to, and then over, the brink of his ability to cope with stress. Eventually he began to drink in order to find relief from the onslaught of his self-imposed stress. His partners noticed his absence from some important meetings, especially in the afternoon. They recognized this as a pattern consistent with problem drinking and insisted that he come to the STRESSCONTROL Center for couseling.

He described his crushing self-imposed standards to me and their effects on him — his migraines, his sleepless nights and his constant dissatisfaction with his own performance.

I asked him to imagine that someone was sitting in the empty chair next to him. I said I would speak on behalf of this imaginary person. "Fred," I said, "you may think you're a good lawyer but you're really not so hot. You don't deserve the reputation you have, and if I were you, I'd stay up nights worrying about when your facade of competence was going to crumble. Rather than status and satisfaction, you deserve only migraine headaches and constant aggravation."

I could see him shifting angrily in his chair, clenching his teeth and gripping the arm of the chair tightly. "What do you feel about what the guy in the chair next to you just said?" Fred exploded, "I could kill the son-of-a-bitch," and then he suddenly smiled realizing that he was talking about his own tyrannical conscience. "You see," I said, "you have an element of your mind that sits in judgement of you — we all have that little critic in our heads. However, your inner critic really forgot that critics can bestow acclaim as well as condemnation. You need to reprogram or reeducate that inner critic of yours to be more in tune with the real facts of your performance. Don't accept the judgement of your inner critic without reflecting on the quality and accuracy of the criticism itself."

Too many people just assume that the rules in their own head that govern their behavior are immutable for all time, whether they work well or cause undue stress and hardship. If you don't like the judgements passed on you by your inner critic, fire him! It's your prerogative to set the rules for your own life in such a way that they help you to cope with stress rather than impose it on you.

There is no state in life to which you can aspire that gives you more freedom than you have now to live your life as you choose. *You're there right now! You have the right to live your own way right now!*

Coordinate the wanting, doing, and judging aspects of your mind to produce results rather than stress.

- *Focus* on your vital needs.
- *Rehearse* constructive solutions and strategies for attaining your goals.
- *Implement* those solutions with a responsible, supportive and reasonable internal critic in operation.

You *can* defeat the stresses that may affect your mind by recognizing the mind's dynamic stability and giving it a rest when that is required. Try meditation rather than alcohol or pills to assist the process of mental relaxation. Learning to put down your mental burdens twice a day through meditation, or even a scheduled rest, can help restore your vitality and energy, making it easier for you to pick up and carry your mental load the rest of the day.

3
Stress and
Your Health

Adelaide's Lament

> *In other words, just from waiting around for that plain little*
> *band of gold,*
> *A person — can develop a cold.*
>
> *You can feed her all day with the Vitamin A and the Bromo*
> *Fizz, —*
> *But the medicine never gets anywhere near where the trouble*
> *is.** *

What a marvelous and perceptive lyric this is when it comes to describing stress and how it affects your health. Adelaide is trapped in a frustrating and, at the same time, gratifying relationship with Nathan Detroit. After years of fruitless courtship, she has dug herself deeply into an emotional rut, having lied to her mother in an effort to reduce the embarrassment of not yet being married.

At the same time, she loves Nathan and so is unwilling to give him an ultimatum which might terminate the relationship. The result is that she lives with ever-diminishing hopes that he will marry her and suffers chronic upper respiratory tract problems as a *direct result* of her frustrations, and also as an *indirect means of coping* with Nathan's indifference through evoking his sympathy for her via her physical symptoms. She tells him poignantly and accurately that the ". . . medicine never gets anywhere near where the trouble is . . ."

All psychosomatic problems have the same three-part make-up as Adelaide's:

1. *Stressful social forces:* The disapproval of family and community of prolonged and non-legally sanctioned male-female cohabitation.

2. *Stressful internal psychological forces:* Adelaide's repeated disappointments, frustration, growing hopelessness and sadness over not yet being married after such a long courtship.

3. *Expressive physical symptoms:* Coughing, wheezing, sneezing, sinus problems, etc. These symptoms are real in the sense that her cold is caused by a viral invasion of her body. In addition, the symptoms are *expressive* in the sense that they make her eyes weep and cause her to be ill, thus evoking Nathan's sympathy and protective feelings.

Stress that causes disease is rarely from one source alone — either social *or* emotional *or* physical. Rather, stress arises usually from all three sources in varying proportions. Adelaide's shame was the strongest disease-causing force and it came from the social sphere. Her own emotional stress was second in importance, causing her to want to weep silently all the time, hence the over-secretion of tears and mucous that blocked her sinuses. Lastly, the disease agent, the virus which floats through the air ready to infect anyone and everyone, found a susceptible victim in Adelaide because of the decrease in her resistance to infection due to chronic stress.

Scientific studies have shown clearly that a person's mind-body reaction can be exactly the same no matter whether the stress comes from the social, psychological or physical spheres.

As you watch the annual Harvard-Yale boat race on the Charles River, you are impressed by the fantastic expenditure of energy of the rowing crew. You watch the boats sliding swiftly through the water, propelled by the powerful rhythmic strokes of the oarsmen, synchronized by the cadence of the coxswain's shouts through his megaphone. "Lucky guy, that coxswain," you think. "He gets the same amount of glory for exercising his vocal cords as do the oarsmen for straining every muscle in their bodies to the limit. Their stress is so much greater than his, right?" Wrong! Oarsmen, coxswain and even the coach back on the dock are under similar levels of stress* in terms of the body's reactions, even though in the case of the oarsmen, physical strain is the chief force; in the coxswain, psychological strain predominates; and in the coach, psychological and perhaps, social forces (his duty to uphold the good reputation of the college) are paramount. When the body's stress hormone levels are checked and blood counts are done to detect white blood cell reactions to stress, oarsmen, coxswain and coach all show severe stress signs — *even before the race begins!* While these severe stress reactions are quickly and harmlessly terminated after the excitement of the race is over, in situations of prolonged social or psychological stress, by contrast, resistance to disease would be impaired over a long period and a physical illness might result. Hence, the wisdom of Adelaide's statement, "the medicine never gets anywhere near where the trouble is." Her disease is caused by the stress of the prolonged courtship more than it is by the Streptococcus bacteria.

The "New" versus the "Old" Medicine

For many years it has been known to the medical profession that every disease is caused by the following sequence of events:

*Hill, S. R. Jr., et al: "Studies on Adrenocortical and Psychological Response to Stress in Man," ARCHIVES OF INTERNAL MEDICINE, 97 (1956): 269–298.

$$\left\{ \begin{array}{c} \text{Lowered} \\ \text{Resistance} \end{array} \right\} + \left\{ \begin{array}{c} \text{Exposure to a} \\ \text{Disease Causing Agent} \end{array} \right\} \longrightarrow \text{Illness}$$

"Old" or traditional medicine emphasized an attack on the disease-causing agent:

- Antibiotics to kill bacteria.
- Purification of the water supply to prevent exposure to harmful bacteria, viruses or chemical toxins.
- Correction of metabolic or endocrine defects which cause the body to function abnormally, thus producing disease (diabetes, hyperthyroidism, etc.)

"Old" or traditional mental health efforts were also aimed at correction and/or elimination of disease-causing agents:

- Traumatic childhood experiences which produced a neurosis were reviewed, relived, and understood through psychoanalysis. This gave the person an opportunity to apply adult intellect to correct buried and influential assumptions originating in the warped childhood experiences.
- Improperly learned responses to emotional conflict (phobias, anxiety neuroses, etc.) were sorted out and restructured through individual and group therapy or their disturbing emotional consequences controlled through tranquilizers and/or antidepressants.

Traditional medicine and psychiatry focused almost exclusively on preventing exposure to or reducing the residual harm from exposure to the disease-causing agent. The techniques used were, and still are, complex, powerful and useful, and require skilled manpower to implement them. The emphasis on *cure* through the use of drugs, surgery or powerful psychological treatments led to a passive role on the part of the patient, who underwent that "cure" at the hands of an "expert." Patients were advised to come in for periodic checkups by the "expert" who could discover the early effects of a disease-producing agent and implement a cure while there was still time. This approach was and still is valid, necessary and not in conflict with an emerging trend in medical circles to a "holistic" or "new" medicine which emphasizes, in addition to traditional techniques, stress control, nutrition, and adequate exercise as means of increasing resistance to disease, thus preventing its occurrence in the first place.

Key features of this approach are as follows:

1. The methods are *safe* and the patient learns how to apply them when needed. (When did you know of anyone who overdosed on biofeedback relaxation therapy or organically grown vegetables?)
2. The objective is *prevention* rather than cure of disease through improving health rather than attacking illness-causing agents.
3. Mind and body are considered indivisible and the emphasis is placed on producing harmony in the three key domains of life — *social, expressive emotional, and physical.*
4. Educational and training methods are used to improve a person's ability to live a healthy lifestyle as contrasted with medical treatment approaches which rely on the doctor's ability to repair the effects of an unhealthy lifestyle.

Some sample cases:

• A bored, assembly-line worker doing a repetitive job in an electronics plant develops arthritis. There is an "old" and a "new" approach to her problem. Which should she choose?
• An air-traffic controller begins to develop high blood levels of substances associated with coronary heart disease — should he look to the "new" or "old" medicine for an answer?
• A woman suffering migraine headaches for thirty years is unable to find much relief through the use of drugs. She

begins to suffer drug side effects and now must even give up
what little benefit the medicines provided. Where shall she
turn?

• A diabetic teenage boy cannot be properly controlled on
insulin and has been frequently brought to the emergency ward
in a coma. His pediatrician is increasingly worried that one day
the ambulance won't get to the hospital on time. What new
method or skill can he apply for his patient's benefit, perhaps
even to save the child's life?

• A young man begins to suffer shortness of breath soon after
the death of his mother. Medical tests are negative for a
detectable disease. He fears he will die in asphyxiation as did
his mother who had congestive heart failure. What is going
on in him — what can help him?

Is "old" medicine the answer? Shall we turn to "new" medicine
to help these clearly distressed patients? The uncertainty abound-
ing in contemporary medicine, both among practitioners and con-
sumers, as to what road will lead to salvation, has spawned many
cults that purport to cure all ills. Many oversold methods which, if
properly restricted and understood would be safe and valid, are
recklessly huckstered by gurus and "preventive medicine"
quacks. Much unfair criticism is leveled at useful methods of care
just because they are "old" and conventional, or simply because
they are "new" and unconventional. Pity the poor layman under
stress, feeling pain, and looking for help, who is faced with an
unprecedented selection of approaches to his or her problem, having no rationale or guidelines to know where to start looking for
help and in what context to place all these promises of "relief."

Let's return to the equation cited earlier to understand how
disease occurs. Perhaps in analyzing the basic mechanism of the
genesis of illness we can find a proper place for all useful techniques and eliminate those that aren't appropriate.

Returning now to our distressed and confused patients we
might suggest the following:

> • For the bored, understimulated, sedentary assembly-line
> worker who is developing arthritis due to, among other
> reasons, inadequate levels of stimulation and activity, we

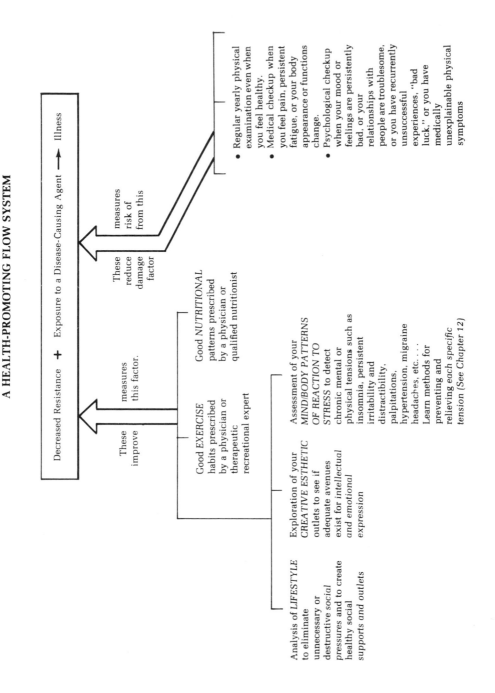

A HEALTH-PROMOTING FLOW SYSTEM

Decreased Resistance **+** Exposure to a Disease-Causing Agent → Illness

These improve

These reduce damage factor

measures this factor.

measures risk of from this

Good EXERCISE habits prescribed by a physician or therapeutic recreational expert

Good NUTRITIONAL patterns prescribed by a physician or qualified nutritionist

Exploration of your CREATIVE ESTHETIC outlets to see if adequate avenues exist for intellectual and emotional expression

Assessment of your MIND/BODY PATTERNS OF REACTION TO STRESS to detect chronic mental or physical tensions such as insomnia, persistent irritability and distractibility, palpitations, hypertension, migraine headaches, etc. . . . Learn methods for preventing and relieving each specific tension (See Chapter 12)

Analysis of LIFESTYLE to eliminate unnecessary or destructive social pressures and to create healthy social supports and outlets

- Regular yearly physical examination even when you feel healthy.
- Medical checkup when you feel pain, persistent fatigue, or your body appearance or functions change.
- Psychological checkup when your mood or feelings are persistently bad, or your relationships with people are troublesome, or you have recurrently unsuccessful experiences, "bad luck," or you have medically unexplainable physical symptoms

might recommend an exercise program on the job that would compensate for the sedentary nature of her work; creative-aesthetic activities to provide needed emotional expression and mental stimulation; relaxation training through the use of biofeedback methods if the arthritis is caused in part or is complicated by chronic muscle tension; and good quality medical care to monitor the effects of all these efforts and to apply pharmacological intervention when necessary.

• For the overpressured air-traffic controller whose heart and circulatory system are beginning to suffer from the stress of his responsibility for so many people's safety, we might recommend: a consultation with a nutritionist to provide a diet that will help reduce cholesterol and other substances in the blood that contribute to coronary artery disease; training in biofeedback relaxation methods to reduce cardiovascular overexertion; as closely supervised medical program including a cardiac stress evaluation to monitor heart functioning and risk factors; and a change in lifestyle to reduce unnecessary social pressures and increase social supports and outlets. Recognizing his need for emotional support, the wife of one air-traffic controller made sure that she acted as family gatekeeper for stressful social and family pressures. She protected his privacy when he was home and bore the lion's share of all social arrangements.

• For the woman suffering migraine headaches and now unable to use her medications, a medically supervised biofeedback relaxation training program can offer up to 80% expected cure rates in appropriate candidates who remain in the training program, and who apply the methods when under stress or just as the migraine "aura" (or warning symptoms) are beginning.

• For the diabetic teenage boy who is difficult to control on insulin, we might review nutrition and exercise patterns to start. Lifestyle social pressures might be examined to determine if the youngster has a confidant with whom he can unload emotional burdens and fears, and who can also provide him valid support and encouragement. In an actual

case, the brother of a young fatherless boy enlisted in the
Navy. This caused so much stress in the child that his
diabetes became difficult to control. Finding him a "big
brother" to replace his real brother helped control his illness.
Medical monitoring of the diabetes should be supplemented
by a psychological checkup to examine whether there are
hidden sources of emotional stress in the youngster's mind
which could provoke instability of his blood sugar.
● For the young man who is short of breath following the
death of his mother from congestive heart failure, a
psychological checkup might reveal emotional factors
underlying his breathing problems. These might be rooted in
guilt feelings that he should have been kinder to his mother
in the last few years before her death. These guilt feelings
produce a need for self-punishment which often takes
the form of mirroring a symptom experienced by the
deceased person. In this case, the shortness of breath
experienced by his mother, who was dying from congestive
heart failure, was taken on by the son in a *self-punitive
identification* with his mother. "I deserve to suffer with her in
the same way as she did, through shortness of breath," he
unconsciously decided. "That would be fitting punishment
for my neglect of her in the years before her death." This
actual case history occurred in my practice and the young
man was cured as a result of psychotherapy which helped
him explore and deal with his guilt feelings without needing
the physical symptom as a means of expressing his
atonement.

As in most complex and technical fields, a combination of the
best "old" and "new" methods, rationally integrated and applied,
offers the individual the best approach to his or her health problems. When we think of the marathon race we are all in — that is,
getting through life from birth to old age in the healthiest possible
way — we can learn a lot from the winning Grand Prix auto racer.
He gives his car the ultimate in good care and periodic inspections to make sure the equipment is always in top shape. He
also handles the equipment with respect — pacing himself rather

than forcing the machine to run at top speed all the time at the risk of blowing his engine. He makes pit stops when necessary, but always *before* his fuel runs out. He respects, admires and cares for his equipment and it, in turn, takes good care of him.

We must learn, like the Grand Prix racer, to give our bodies, minds, habits and lifestyles periodic inspections. We must pace ourselves and come in for a rest break before our fuel runs out. Preventive maintenance and careful handling of the body and mind will get us through the grand prix of life with comfort, confidence and health. Reckless and wasteful abuse of mind and body will put us at risk of dangerous breakdowns in our health.

Pain and Illness as a Means of Self-Expression and/or Reaction to Environmental Stress

If Adelaide caught *la grippe* in part because of social pressures and sanctions against common-law relationships, and if a rowing coach can spew stress hormones into his bloodstream as a reaction to feeling duty-bound to uphold the reputation of his college (and perhaps preserve his job), then where do we draw the line between society, the mind, and the body? The fact is, we cannot separate these domains. They continuously interact irrespective of the species studied.

Put mice and rats in overcrowded quarters and they show a decrease in fertility.* The same reduced fertility has been found when hens are overcrowded. Put mice who are unfamiliar with one another together in one cage and abnormal changes in brain chemistry are produced as a direct result.‡ The mind, body and social environment are in a constant game of ping-pong with one system slamming the stress ball into the other system's court and vice versa. The effects of stress in any domain have impact

*Christian, J. J., "A Review of the Endocrine Responses in Rats and Mice to Increase in Population Size Including Delayed Effects on Offspring," NAVAL MED. RES. INST. (Aug. 6, 1957), pp. 443–462.
‡Bliss, E. L., Ailion, J., "Response of Neurogenic Amines to Aggregation and Strangers," J. PHARMACOL. EXP. THER., 168 (1969): 258–263.

everywhere else. Emotions can cause physical changes. Social influences have mind and body effects. A physical injury has social and psychological consequences, and so on. When we consider stress and health, it is a case of "mind over matter" since there is no way of restricting the influences one system has upon another.

While mind, body and social forces continuously interact in an infinite number of combinations, several patterns of interactions can be usefully categorized.

THE EFFECTS OF MENTAL STIMULATION ON YOUR HEALTH

We all know from personal experience that it is almost worse than being overworked on a job to be underutilized and bored. Recently, a scientific study of people in work settings confirmed this belief, showing that disease/risk factors are highest when people experience either a lack or an excess of stimulation in their jobs: being either underworked or overworked is unhealthy; ambiguity or extreme rigidity in relation to work tasks increases disease/risk factors; extreme role conflict or very little responsibility seems to cause health hazards to employees.* It appears that the human mind needs an optimum dose of activity, responsibility, aggravation and social structure in order to operate with maximum effectiveness and in good health. If you become ill, you may well wish to analyze your work setting according to the above disease/risk factors to see if your "work is making you sick," as you have, perhaps, long suspected.

IS MY PAIN REAL OR IMAGINARY?

Many people, upon hearing the term "psychosomatic," immediately equate it with a person faking illness for attention or sympathy. On the contrary, psychosomatic illness is *real* illness both to the mind and the body. What makes it "psychosomatic"

*Weiman, Clinton G., "A Study of Occupational Stressor and the Incidence of Disease Risk," JOURNAL OF OCCUPATIONAL MEDICINE 19, no. 2 (Feb. 1977), pp. 119–122.

is the prominent role played in its development by social and emotional forces, as contrasted to "real" illness caused, for example, by being run over by a steamroller or the invasion of the body by the measles virus. In these cases, we rarely invoke the notion of causative social and psychological forces because the physical manifestations are so blatant and well known. You won't get far asking, "I wonder if Bill's problems at home made him more careless and caused him to step in front of the steamroller." Or "Johnny got the measles . . . I wonder if his poor report card had anything to do with lowering his resistance?"

Nevertheless, all accidents require a merging of physical circumstances and people who find their way into those events. My own experiences with car accidents have convinced me that rushing to a meeting with people I detested *had* to have played a role in running my BMW smack into a ten-ton gravel truck. Or once, when going to my psychoanalyst's to discuss a painful and recurring interpersonal problem for which I could find no solution, I avoided that necessity by "accidentally" ramming another car from the rear. For many people, accidents are just waiting to happen. I have been among the accident prone on several occasions, always due to the stresses of my emotional and social environment.

Many of the pains we experience replicate pains we have experienced at other times or pains that people we know have suffered. I have already described the phenomenon of *self-punitive identification* — the young man who punished himself for neglecting his mother by unconsciously deciding to incorporate into his life her shortness of breath. If you checked his respirations with a special lung capacity machine, it would have shown more labored respiration than normal. He had true respiratory distress at the level of the work done by his chest muscles and diaphragm, even though his lungs and circulation were normal and thus he, in contrast to his dying mother, got enough oxygen into his system. His respiratory distress was his way of punishing himself for his failure to show his mother adequate consideration before her death and was not relieved until he had expressed his anger at her in one of our therapy sessions. This proved to be the root cause of his reluctance to be near her in her old age.

Many people suffer recapitulations of symptoms they have had in earlier life. One woman developed pains in her abdomen which extensive medical investigation proved were not due to physical disease. In therapy, we discovered that, as a child, she actually had had an abdominal disease due to a malformation of her intestines from birth. She was a neglected child in every other sphere of life. Her brother outperformed her scholastically. Her younger sister received all the attention that "the baby of the family" usually commands. And yet, when her abdominal pains started up, life in the family came to a halt and her parents rushed around frantically, calling her doctor, bringing her medications and brushing the other children's needs aside in favor of caring for her. Eventually, the intestinal problem was successfully corrected through surgery. She grew into adulthood, symptom-free following the corrective operation.

As an adult, when she encountered neglect by her husband and, later, by her grown children, she developed severe abdominal pains — carbon copies of the pains from her childhood. The impact of her pains on her family was also identical. Life revolved around catering to her needs as long as the pain persisted. Eventually, through a combination of individual and family psychotherapy, she learned to obtain consideration from others in less alarming and more comfortable ways. The pains stopped and never recurred. In this case, her pains really had a message in them: "I want love, consideration and my fair share of attention." When she learned how to verbalize and enact this request in her relationships with family members, this message was transferred back from the physical to the interpersonal realm of expression, where it belonged.

Perhaps the most difficult form of psychosomatic illness to understand is that in which no seeming connection exists between emotional and social stresses and the illness itself. There appears to be no logical connection or even any symbolic connection between the emotion and the illness in the case of emotional tension and gastric or duodenal ulcers; between guilt feelings and thrombophlebitis; between hidden rage and high blood pressure; between anger at a domineering, controlling parent and ulcerative colitis. These are only a few of many psychosomatic conditions that patients steadfastly refuse to acknowledge as having any roots except in physical or genetic-hereditary factors. "All of my family is ulcer-prone. Don't tell me it has anything to do with the way I live," said one patient of mine. True enough, the tendency to oversecrete stomach acid and enzymes is hereditary, but it takes social and emotional stresses, usually unfulfilled desires, to trigger off the gastric secretions. The person craves satisfaction; the stomach lining, reacting to a reflex present since infancy, prepares itself for a satisfying feeding; and the person who, due to heredity, oversecretes stomach acid and enzymes, begins to digest his own stomach lining. This sequence causes stomach and duodenal ulcers and has all three of the components of any psychosomatic illness:

1. *Social forces* — Inadequate satisfaction for the individual (in this case, a failing business).
2. *Emotional forces* — Feelings of frustration, and a craving for satisfaction.
3. *Physical reactions* — Outpouring of stomach acid and enzymes in a genetically predisposed stomach lining.

Since we can't change heredity once it has endowed us with a vulnerable stomach lining, we can either eliminate the stomach through surgery, decrease the flow of or neutralize the acid through medicines and antacids, or ameliorate the destructive social and emotional forces causing the mismatch between the person's needs and his capacity to satisfy them. A stress control approach to this problem emphasized:

1. Increasing the patient's coping skills to satisfy his needs. (In this case, a capable business consultant did a great deal of good.)
2. Assessing his needs to see if they were appropriate and realistic. (This patient couldn't wait to be a millionaire as was his brother-in-law.) Then, scaling down his demands to realizable levels, he recognized what was realistically possible in the foreseeable future.
3. Reducing the time pressure on himself for satisfying

these needs. (Millions aren't made in weeks or months — it takes a total successful business career to achieve this goal.)

The stress control formula was useful in reminding him what to do to solve the problem:

- *Reduce* the complexity or number of tasks confronting you (eliminate unrealistic requirements).
- *Reduce* the time pressure to complete these tasks.
- *Increase* coping capacity through education or psychotherapy (need-satisfying abilities).

Take the case of an attractive middle-aged woman whose husband died suddenly. She was beset by guilt feelings which were especially intense in her situation because her husband had been a selfish man and she realized his death was a golden opportunity for her to redesign her life to her own benefit after years of frustration and deprivation. So repugnant was the thought that his death was actually "good luck" for her, that she restricted her social life severely in order not to profit from this "good luck" which would have exacerbated her over-whelming guilt feelings. Three months after his death, she developed a serious case of thrombophlebitis. When I suggested that it had an emotional stress dimension to it, she recoiled and resisted. Finally, I asked her to consider the case of former President Richard Nixon who also suffered from thrombophlebitis. "What feelings do you suppose he had when under fire from inside his own party and from adversaries all around him?" "Anger, guilt feelings, and also sadness over the loss of his good reputation," she replied.

"If I spoke out loud the effect on you of your husband's death, I would have to say, 'Good riddance.' What would that make you feel — anger? — guilt feelings? — a fear that you would lose your good reputation if people knew you wished your husband dead?" She got the message and realized her most significant stresses were in her own mixed emotional reactions to her husband's death. She began to return to the normal life of an attractive widow and her guilt feelings diminished and then disappeared. Her thrombophlebitis improved and then disappeared, too, just as the former president's did when he was removed as the focal point of intense accusations by his peers.

No matter how many times I illustrate to patients the connection between social stress, its emotional counterparts and the consequent physical reactions produced, people vigorously resist this notion. Yet, no one I have ever met will question the connection between social humiliation, the emotional reaction of shame, and the dilatation of facial skin blood vessels we call blushing. It seems that as long as the physical reaction is obvious — as with an embarrassed blush — and it comes at the same time as we recognize the social and emotional stresses that produced it, we can accept the causal connections. However, in the case of internal and, therefore, invisible "blushes," we are skeptical about their social and emotional connections.

We accept scatological references as a natural expression of anger and frustration. "Aw, shit, don't tell me you did it again." "When the boss sees this, the shit will really hit the fan." "Don't dump your shit on me, man." When the stubborn child is overpowered by a domineering parent, we accept the fact that he will either hold back excreting his feces, or deposit them in some inconvenient place at some inconvenient time. Yet, when an ulcerative colitis patient is first told to seek psychotherapy because of the "psychological factors" involved in his or her condition, the reaction is frequently negative. People are resistant to the idea that a hyperactive bowel could in any way be connected with a response to overpowering social or interpersonal forces. When such a person is under stress, however, "the shit" really does "hit the fan," and the chronically and severely overworked colon begins to ulcerate.

Pain and illness are means of self-expression and reactions to environmental stress. We must learn to use these important signals from our bodies rather than to petulantly and stubbornly ignore them.

First, we must *focus* on what the body signal might be revealing: Is it a message telling me and the world how frustrated I am with my husband or wife? Is it a "blush" in one of my internal organs which has been triggered into destructive overwork by anger or an unfulfilled need? Is it a sign of a too harsh internal critic making me feel excessively guilty and causing concurrent physical distress?

Next, we must *rehearse* positive solutions to the problem. We must learn effective verbal and emotional ways to convey what the body is trying to communicate. We must redesign relationships so that inherent destructive social and emotional forces are eliminated.

Finally, we must learn to consistently and appropriately *implement* the new constructive behavior, be it more effective emotional and verbal communication, better household or business management, or turning to friends for support when needed, instead of shunning them.

Good stress control habits and practices can improve resistance to illness. Combined with good medical care, these preventive measures can reduce in severity and even eliminate many stress-related diseases from our lives.

4
Stressful Emotions and What to Do about Them

If God Didn't Want Man to Cry, He Wouldn't Have Given Him Tears

There is no aspect of our creation in which nature has left us so incomplete as in our emotional reactions. We compound nature's flaws by our own deliberate self-deception through distorting the awareness and expression of our emotions.

When it comes to physical endangerment, nature has provided us with a quick and efficient combination of sensations and reflex actions. Put your hand on a hot stove and so quick and efficient is your natural reaction of physical self-preservation that you will jerk your hand away before the danger signal reaches your mind: "hot stove — *beware* — *ouch!*"

This is not the case at all with emotions. Let an emotion rise to the surface of your consciousness and you might react, "There's no reason for me to feel depressed. I'd better just try to forget about it, get it out of my mind. Maybe if I get busy with something I'll forget about the depressed feelings." In the domain of emotional self-preservation, the reflex action is to disregard the warning signal — the emotional reaction — and try to ward it off or suppress it if it persists. Small wonder, then, that the causes giving rise to these emotions remain hidden, often growing in severity and number. Finally, a person is overwhelmed by the constant cacophony of emotional warning signals and may need to turn off the entire alarm system with tranquilizers and/or alcohol. Nature did not do herself proud when it came to emotions as a self-preserving signal system. Emotional signals are imprecise, leaving us dangling in panic or despair when they are evoked, and not leading to a crisp and efficient reaction of self-preservation as is the case with sensations of physical danger. We must learn to correct nature's deficient design of our emotional warning system. We need to learn how to decipher and react to emotional messages that alert us that something has gone wrong.

Everyone has had many experiences that convincingly demonstrate how emotions can interfere with life. Do you remember the time you forgot your lines in the school play because you were too nervous? Or the time everyone chuckled at your awkwardness as you made a Freudian slip at a party, revealing a true but buried feeling about your husband? "I'll *prevent* him with the opportunity to relax whenever he needs to," you said, when you really wanted to say, "*present*." You thus revealed that you have mixed feelings about the amount or type of your husband's leisure activities.

Emotions do tend to insert themselves in awkward places at inopportune times. Rather than regard them as potentially important though annoying sources of information, we try to deny, camouflage, modify or dilute their message content. "I'm sort of upset at what you did," you say, to soften your rage at being hurt by someone's neglect. "I'm disappointed in you," you say when you really feel furious. "The kids are really getting to me," you tell your husband, when you really believe that the problem is that your husband isn't giving you any support in disciplining the children. We take nature's already garbled emotional warning signals and further confuse ourselves by changing their source or direction, changing their quality and stifling or disguising their expression. Sometimes we even question the existence of an obvious emotion because there is no apparent reason to justify its existence or because it has no clear and practical use at the moment. "You're really upset," you tell your friend. "No, I'm not," he angrily replies. "And what good is being upset going to do for me anyway?" he adds.

There is as much logic to this position as there would be for someone to refuse to acknowledge the presence of the moon orbiting the earth. "Look, *you* may see something up there in the sky but *I don't!* Anyway, what good would it do me it I saw what you call 'a moon'? Does it do me any good to see it? I mean, if nature had put a giant exhaust fan in the sky to get rid of air pollution, then I'd acknowledge its presence, but what good is a pile of rocks in outer space?"

Sound absurd? It's no more off the wall than denying the existence of your emotions just because you can't, for the moment, make practical use out of them. If watched and tracked, emotions will ultimately lead you to the most vital areas requiring attention in your life: Your hidden needs, and the deficiencies requiring repair in your relationships with people.

Dealing with Emotions on the Installment Plan

Because emotions can be disruptive to smooth functioning in life or even, at the extreme, prevent functioning at all, nature has endowed us with a way of filtering emotions out of consciousness, allowing only small doses of emotion to enter awareness at any given time. These dimly perceived emotions call attention to important problems at an early stage of their development, giving us an opportunity to apply solutions while our energy level is highest and the problems giving rise to the emotions are still within manageable proportions. Even when faced with a severe problem, nature's filtering system, if operating properly, lets us handle the emotions in installments.

A man was involved in a bad car accident in which his wife and child were seriously injured. When I talked to him on the scene, he was relatively composed, considering the circumstances. Even though he was crying and extremely worried, he launched a series of protective actions, making sure the police phoned ahead to the hospital to ready the emergency room staff for the arrival of his injured wife and child. He also made sure that a call was put in for a plastic surgeon as his daughter had sustained serious facial lacerations. He functioned efficiently in this way until he got home that evening. Only then did he begin to react more intensely with sorrow and anger. Further installments of emotions were experienced in his dreams. He dreamed repeatedly of his fears and memories of the moment of impact which he had brushed from his conscious mind during the day. This day-by-day and night-by-night reliving of the car accident went on for weeks as his mind slowly digested the massively frightening experience morsel by morsel. Eventually, his nightmares ceased and his mental preoccupation with the accident during waking hours subsided. His thoughts about his wife's and daughter's well-being, the car accident and all the memories surrounding it assumed normal proportions. Nature had permitted him to function effectively during the crisis and to defer paying his emotional dues until later. He then coped with the agony of the experience piecemeal over several weeks. This mind-saving and lifesaving filtering system with which we have been provided can easily be abused. Many people exposed to overpowering emotional circumstances put off paying the emotional price and then try to keep from ever dealing with the emotions at all.

A woman I treated had been raped some years back. She decided not to press charges and just forget the whole thing, vowing never again to walk alone through the dimly lit company parking lot. She succeeded in keeping the rape experience from bothering her for several years until she and her boyfriend began having sex. She could not achieve orgasm and was so emotionally bland during lovemaking that he questioned her about his own adequacy as a sex partner. "I don't know why but no matter what I do, I can't ever turn you on," he said, ashamed of his performance. Her efforts to console and encourage him were unsuccessful as, in his mind, actions spoke louder than words. He was convinced that she didn't care for him and was ready to break off the relationship. In order to prevent this from occurring, she confessed that no man had ever been able to turn her on since the rape. "Something went dead inside. I get to a point just short of climax and then I just shut down emotionally," she painfully revealed. Her boyfriend was understanding, but not reassured, and broke off the relationship, reaching out for women he could please sexually and at the same time who would repair the injury to his confidence.

After several years of therapy, my patient was finally able to relive the shame, anguish, panic and rage associated with the rape. After having unlocked the mental shackles constricting these feelings, she was able to free up her sexual desire again and her ability to enjoy sex to orgasm was restored.

Emotional dues are best paid promptly in convenient install-ments. Otherwise, like any form of debt, the "compound interest" makes the resolution of the emotional problem far more difficult. Over time, more and more of your energy is expended by the need to keep the emotion hidden. Finally you are forced to deal with it anyway, but you now have a minimum of energy with which to confront an old, neglected problem, compounded by feelings of fear and hopelessness. Prompt attention to emotional signals al-lows you to face with maximum energy, new problems not yet worked into your way of life. You wouldn't neglect the pain signals coming from the hand you accidently placed on a hot radiator. Your hand would fry or be seriously burned. Nature un-fortunately has not given you a similar imperative need to track down and remove causes of emotional pain. However, the damage potential is just as great if you don't react quickly and effectively. You *can* correct nature's deficiency by using your own common sense. When an emotional warning sounds, pay attention to it and try to track down and cope with its source as soon as possible.

The Three Chief Varieties of Emotional Camouflage and How They Foul Up Communication and Problem Solving

Most people evolve mental mechanisms for dealing with trou-bling or unacceptable emotions. Like a code, emotions are au-tomatically translated into unintelligible symbols. As soon as the raw emotion is encoded, an immediate stress is reduced as the mind no longer feels the pain produced by the intense emotion. Unfortunately, since nobody understands the code, communica-tions with people are impaired. The person hiding emotions through the use of this camouflage may eventually lose touch with his or her own genuine feelings and believe the code to be the true message. It becomes impossible to search for important needs within the self or within a relationship when a person's emotions have been converted to an unintelligible code. Consequently, long-term stress is increased.

The three coding systems are as follows:

1. *DIRECT* messages are converted to *DISPLACED* messages. The person fearing the reaction of others to his or her emotions redirects the emotions to safe targets.

One woman, chronically disappointed with her husband as a lover and wage-earner, could not express these feelings directly to him. She feared he would lose even more confidence in himself and perhaps give up trying in one or both spheres. Over the years, she displaced her disappointments to her children, complaining about *their* inadequate scholastic performance, and *their* lack of sufficient gratitude, given the magnitude of her sacrifices on their behalf. So unremitting and unrealistic was her disappointment in the children that even when they performed well, there was still a complaint from her on some score.

The oldest child eventually rebelled and was brought in for treatment. It became apparent that her disappointment in him was redirected from its original destination, her husband. I worked with the whole family to bring this pattern to light and the children were the first to acknowledge how they "always caught it from Mom when she was actually upset with Dad." Her husband quickly responded, refusing to let her scapegoat the children any longer for complaints that were meant for him. "I'm a man. I can take it. You've treated me this way for years — like a kid, never wanting to bother me or worry me. Don't you think I too have been upset about my own inability to earn more money? If we can get together and discuss problems like this, maybe we'll come out with the answers. But, please stop dumping on the kids to protect my 'fragile' feelings."

Emotions can be *displaced* to safe targets. You need to examine your emotional communication pattern to see if you are saying what you feel to the right person. It's obvious that to solve an interpersonal problem the emotional communication must be DIRECT to the person and not to a "safe" surrogate.

2. CLEAR messages are converted to MASKED messages. The person, fearing a specific emotion, converts it to another emotion that he can express more comfortably.

If you fear LOVE, you say, "I admire and respect you."

If you fear RAGE, you say, "I can't understand why you would do this to me — I'm so disappointed in you."

If you fear SHAME, you say, "You bastard, look at what you got me into. Do you want to make an ass out of me by your stupidity?"

If you fear GUILT, you say, "He deserved what he got — it's survival of the fittest you know."

If you fear SADNESS, you say, "They did this to me. If it wasn't for your relatives, I wouldn't be having this trouble."

- LOVE becomes RESPECT.
- RAGE becomes DISAPPOINTMENT.
- SHAME becomes DISPARAGEMENT of others.
- GUILT becomes a NECESSITY for survival.
- SADNESS becomes PARANOIA.

As long as emotional messages are masked, their solution is impossible. If you love me, tell me, so that I can love you back if I choose. If you hate me, tell me, so that I might change my ways if you mean something to me. If you feel humiliated, don't disparage me, driving off any encouragement I might be able to offer you.

Emotions must be UNMASKED and made CLEAR so that their impact and meaning will not be misunderstood, leading to misdirected responses.

3. VERBAL messages are converted to NONVERBAL messages. We all express emotions through body language — the most common form of nonverbal emotional expression. Other important varieties exist as well.

Selective inattention or interruptions can convey to a person that what he has to say is unimportant to you.

The *time sequence* of a remark might reveal as much or more than its content. "We'd better be getting home soon. We told the babysitter we would be home by 1 a.m.," is a remark that, when inserted just after your wife captures the interest of the party with her sense of humor and charm, tells her that you resent her and feel competitive or inferior to her. Sometimes *failure to respond* when a response is called for conveys a chilling message of rage.

In all cases where messages are nonverbally sent, their emotional content should be expressed by the recipient:

> "Look, Frank, I was good enough not to cause a commotion in front of the children, but when I made an important point to them at dinner and you sat there in silence and then said, 'Pass the salad, Jenny,' I felt like dumping it on your head. You were basically conveying, 'Don't pay attention to your mother or take her too seriously. She's good for making salads but not for making important decisions. That's my domain.' "

Very often, people use a combination of all three codes at once, ensuring that no one, including themselves, will ever detect their hidden emotions. Recently, a man I was treating put his fist through the bedroom wall following an argument with his wife over their son's school failure. He was enraged at her defense of the boy whom, she claimed, was "trying his hardest." After spending several hours with the couple, I was able to decipher the code.

The *RAGE* originated in *SADNESS*. Father was disappointed with his own career. He had just been given a lateral transfer, a sure sign that his trip up the ladder of success was grinding to a halt. The *SADNESS*, originating in his own life, was masked as *RAGE*, and displaced to his wife. His career frustration was communicated nonverbally, as he poked his fist through a wall in his desperation and inability to punch his way through the obstacles preventing him from further career advancement. He was much better off when his pain was decoded and his wife expressed her love for him, even though he would never be president of his company.

To improve communication and reduce emotional stress, you must learn to decode your own emotional communications and those of others.

- Make *DISPLACED* messages *DIRECT*.
- Make *MASKED* messages *CLEAR*.
- Make *NONVERBAL* messages *VERBAL*.

The Fearsome Foursome — Depression, Anxiety, Guilt Feelings and Feelings of Inadequacy.

In my experience as a psychiatrist, the emotions that create and intensify stress more than any others are depression, anxiety, guilt feelings and feelings of inadequacy. I suspect that it is the helplessness associated with these emotions and the resultant undermining of effective coping efforts that accounts for their stress-intensifying nature. An angry person can still feel and be effective in coping with stress. Love doesn't necessarily prevent anyone from solving problems or being assertive and effective. But depression and optimism are antagonistic entities. Anxiety and confidence rarely go together. Guilt feelings don't engender energy and success strivings. And feelings of inadequacy produce unproductive withdrawal, or rash, impulsive, and usually unsuccessful action to temporarily inflate self-esteem. The fearsome foursome of emotions generally have a paralytic effect on the coping mechanisms we use to deal with these stressful situations. Using a stress control approach you can improve your ability to cope with these stress-intensifying emotions.

- *FOCUSING* on the root cause of the emotion is the first step.
- Next, you must *REHEARSE POSITIVE SOLUTIONS*.
- Finally, you must *IMPLEMENT* these solutions.

DEPRESSION AND WHAT YOU CAN DO ABOUT IT

No matter how varied its manifestations, depression is always caused by a *deficit* in your life. You may have just experienced an actual loss. Or some recent event reminded you of a long abandoned hope never fulfilled. Alternately, an aspiration for future gain may suddenly have appeared futile. In all cases, you feel depressed because of a *deficit* in your life. Frequently, the void is deeply buried, only symbolically or peripherally connected with the triggering event.

Recently a patient of mine became severely depressed because he didn't receive the amount of pay raise he had expected. Since he was independently wealthy, he knew the money couldn't be central to his needs. He *focused* on deficits he had felt in his life and came up with the realization that his father never accorded him any recognition for his achievements. The meager pay raise stimulated this old wound and he became depressed. Having identified the source of his depression, he contemplated positive solutions to his need for recognition. He realized that outside of his work, there were no areas of life that meant much to him. He had put all his eggs in one basket as far as recognition was concerned and was thus exceedingly vulnerable to tiny setbacks at work. He then *rehearsed* ways of coping: trying for more recognition socially by investing more time with friends; diversifying his one-track life by adding a major hobby, and also through greater involvement in philanthropic work. Finally, he *implemented* these solutions and, in the main, was successful. He received greater amounts of recognition outside of work, he received it more regularly and eventually his depression was resolved.

Depression equals *deficit!* Remember this and you will be able to unravel and overcome your depressions.

Frequently, several members of a family play depressive dominoes. Consider the case of two brothers, one twenty-one, and one sixteen, the latter my patient.

The older brother could never live up to his rigid, depressed father's ideals for him. He suffered recurrent depressions and made several suicide attempts, finally succeeding. His younger brother was devastated at the loss of his brother and closest confidant. Previously an excellent scholar and socially outgoing, he withdrew from his peers and eventually stopped attending school due to a host of physical complaints he suffered each morning.

The depressive chain reaction was as follows:

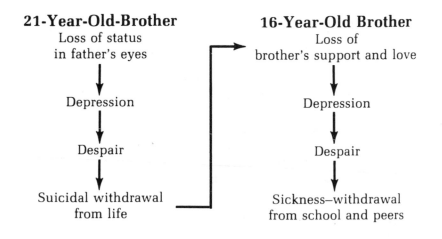

We finally successfully interrupted the chain reaction of *Deficit → Depression → Withdrawal,* by showing the 16-year-old that he could *REPLACE AND REPAIR* his loss. In place of his brother as a confidant, he had me, and later a good friend of his. The withdrawal, he realized, only intensified the effect of the deficit in his life. He learned to find alternative sources for satisfying the needs his brother had so amply filled for him.

The lesson he learned was:

- *Depression* is caused by a *Deficit.*
- The solution to depression is to *replace* and *repair* the lost person, function, or need.

ANXIETY AND WHAT YOU CAN DO ABOUT IT

"You have nothing to fear but fear itself," were the rousing words of Franklin Delano Roosevelt to a despondent nation during the Great Depression.

Succinctly, this sums up why anxiety can produce such overwhelming stress in afflicted people. In its beginnings, anxiety is a mind-saving signal, telling you always that there exists an inner hidden conflict or emotion which, if unattended, will cause you grave problems. Most people don't make this connection, however. They regard the anxiety signal as *the problem itself* and become fearful that they are losing control over their emotions, or even losing their minds. Fear breeds more fear. Anxiety incubates in anxiety. Eventually, the reverberating anxiety circuit intensifies the stress to overwhelming degrees. The person feels doom is near; hyperventilation or sighing respirations — neither of which satisfy the air hunger — get out of hand and the anxious person begins to panic. Palpitations may be added to the picture, convincing the person that a heart attack is underway. Once the cycle gets out of hand, very little except medications like Valium or phenothiazines (Thorazine, Mellaril, etc.) will stop its destructive progression to a temporary emotional breakdown.

By remembering that anxiety in the beginning is an important warning signal, a patient of mine learned to control his anxiety through understanding and resolving its root cause. He was a certified public accountant in partnership with another accountant. His partner was professionally capable and unemotional. For years they had operated effectively as partners, my patient attributing greater feelings of consideration and loyalty to his partner than actually existed . When his partner began to seriously consider dissolving the partnership to move to California, my patient suffered his first of several anxiety attacks. His partner's contemplation of a move for his own good, shattered my patient's long-held but never fully recognized dependency on the man.

"I didn't realize how much of my life was wrapped up in looking to Bill for fatherly protection. When he decided to leave, I must have had a double jolt — one, realizing how dependent upon him I had gotten, and two, being ashamed and not wanting to admit this to myself." At first, my patient did not make the connection when the anxiety signal alerted him to this buried conflict. Instead, he reacted with increasing reverberations of anxiety until the stress was unbearable and overpowering.

Through therapy, he learned to recognize the roots of his anxiety, and was then able to FOCUS on detecting dependency issues when alerted by the anxiety signal. He could then mentally REHEARSE effective measures to deal with his dependency needs — either by trying to satisfy them in appropriate ways with his wife in a mutually interdependent relationship, or with senior colleagues; or by striving for greater self-sufficiency if attainable. He IMPLEMENTED the solution to his anxiety problems as follows:

ANXIETY SIGNAL

↓

FOCUS MY SEARCH ON THREATS TO
MY SECURITY — REVEAL TO MYSELF
DEPENDENCY ISSUES IN MY LIFE

↓

REHEARSE MENTALLY WAYS TO
IMPROVE SECURITY OR TO SECURE
APPROPRIATE HELP FROM OTHERS

↓

IMPLEMENT SOLUTIONS, ESPECIALLY
WHEN ANXIETY SIGNALS BEGIN

GUILT AND INADEQUACY FEELINGS AND WHAT YOU CAN DO ABOUT THEM

If you remember the Ten commandments, you will recall that they were divided into two classes of request:

THOU SHALT
THOU SHALT NOT

The standards of morality of the Ten Commandments resemble in structure the internal yardstick we use to measure our thoughts and behavior and their impact on the world.

In all of us there resides a complex inner legislature that spells out what we must do to be O.K. *(thou shalt)*; and what we must refrain from doing to be O.K. *(thou shalt not)*. We constantly measure and compare all our thoughts, actions and their results against this inner yardstick and evaluate the discrepancy between the prescribed ideal standard and our actual performance. Commit a *thou shalt not* act, and you feel immediate guilt, a sharp reminder of your transgression as assessed by the inner standards. Fail to act adequately in a situation where the inner legislature demands that *thou shalt* act successfully, you feel inadequate and ashamed of yourself. To feel O.K., you must obey all the *thou shalt* and *thou shalt not* commandments etched in your conscience. Otherwise, the penalties are shame and guilt respectively.

The existence in the mind of an unreasonable set of internal standards can create a stress spiral of serious proportions. You may never be able to satisfy all, or even a small portion, of the *thou shalts* in your mind. Or, you may have such an overdose of *thou shalt nots* in your conscience, that any slight move to the left or right provokes guilt feelings. You get into a *no-win* situation, always plagued by self-doubt and guilt. What is worse, a reverberating circuit can get started in which guilt and shame aggravate each other.

Guilt feelings usually cause people to slow down or stop what they are doing. "I'm wrong, I know I'm wrong. I was too assertive and I'm sorry. I won't do it again," the guilty mind promises itself as it slows or shuts down coping operations.

Feelings of inadequacy produce the opposite result. "I've got to hurry up and be a winner; I can't stand losing any more," says the mind suffering feelings of inadequacy. Too often, a gamble or an impulsive action results, causing more failure and guilt feelings. A cycle is generated as follows:

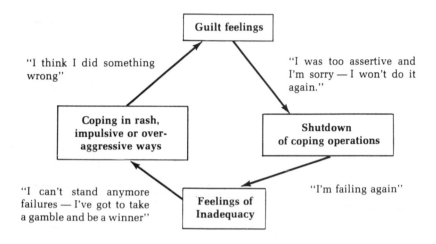

To prevent a destructive cycle from developing and imposing enormous stress upon all your thoughts and actions, you must learn to stand aside from guilt and inadequacy feelings and assess them objectively.

"I feel guilty. What crime did I commit?" If you cannot find a serious moral or ethical infraction, the guilt and its source should be discounted.

"I feel inadequate. By what standards (or by whose standards) have I failed?" If you are O.K. objectively, drop the *thou shalt* whip and refuse to pick it up to flagellate yourself in order to meet someone else's standards or to meet the unrealistic one's you yourself have set.

Dealing effectively with the fearsome foursome of emotions can relieve much stress in your life. Using stress control formulas can assist you in handling these potentially brutal emotions.

• *Reduce* the quantity and complexity of the tasks confronting you. Deal with your emotions when you first feel them. Don't let them accumulate, sapping your energy, leading to a face-off between an aggregate of powerful emotions and a drained, hopeless and frustrated mind. By tracking your emotions to their roots, you will discover important needs that must be attended to and relationships that, if improved, will be more productive and satisfying.

• *Reduce* the time pressure on you for completing the task. Nature's filtering system will hand you emotions on a reasonable installment plan. Don't go overboard trying to psychoanalyze yourself, at the one extreme, or defer indefinitely dealing with an emotion when it becomes apparent, at the other extreme. If you don't deal with emotions piecemeal, you will have to deal with them in a single dose. You may not have sufficient time or energy to cope adequately with long-neglected or denied emotions that burst out all at once in a crisis.

• *Increase* your ability to cope with emotion by learning to *focus* on its roots, *rehearsing* positive solutions for the needs revealed, and then *implementing* these solutions in a hopeful, practical and efficient way. Dreamers are wonderful people. They inspire you to explore your feelings with unprecedented freedom. Be a dreamer when it comes to contemplating solutions to emotional problems. Then be hardnosed and practical when you must implement a solution. If you are depressed, try to find and repair the deficit in your life. If you can't do this, compensate yourself in some other way. That's better than remaining in a depression for too long a time. If you are anxious and can't find the source, don't be heroic. Take a tranquilizer to prevent a runaway cycle of ever-intensifying panic. You can wait until tomorrow, if necessary, to find the exact source of your anxiety. If you are beset by guilt and inadequacy feelings, reset the standards and rules in your mind so that they make life more livable and less stressful.

You *can* do something about stressful emotions if you

remember they are messengers originating in your needs and relationships, sent to your mind. Don't attack or criticize the messenger as the ancient Greeks did when the the message received was unpleasant. Instead, track the emotion until it leads you to its vital warning. Once you know what the job is that needs to be done, you will cope effectively and confidently. Learn to reverse the *displacement, masking* and *nonverbal conversions* of emotions and you will communicate in an effective and authentic manner that will immeasurably reduce emotional stress in your life.

5
The Stresses of
Self-Development

*I'm Prepared to Fight to Defend My Right
to Be a Pacifist*

As paradoxical as it may sound, people are often required to fight to defend their rights to a peaceful, harmonious and satisfying life. Countries, even those professing and practicing pacifism, do a quick turnaround when their own borders are attacked. In recent history, India — homeland of passive resistance, proponent of international pacifism, and exporter of meditation methods, gurus and assorted philosophies of inner peace — has twice gone to war with its neighbors, Pakistan and China, when it felt its vital interests threatened. The late Prime Minister Nehru remarked matter-of-factly, when questioned about his country's surprising bellicosity, "We are pacifists *except at our own borders.*" So, too, must individuals seeking to fulfill their own potential learn to be pacifists except at their own borders. We must define the boundaries of our life space, make sure that this is communicated clearly and directly to those around us, and then be prepared to defend our own borders through assertiveness. Only through maintaining the integrity of your own life space can you develop your potential with a minimum of destructive stress. Unfortunately, nature has left us with some serious imperfections that require repair if we are to succeed in our quest for rewarding self-development.

We all begin life with an undefined, unbounded personal

awareness. The infant cannot distinguish the inner pain of hunger from the outer world of people and things. Consequently, when feeling hunger pangs, the infant's mind confuses the inner discomfort with the entire world around him and he sees pain coming from every person and thing in his life. Fear and panic develop and build, feeding on themselves as the infant becomes frightened of its own screams and the labored respirations that accompany the terror. You arrive with bottle in hand and stuff the nipple into a trembling, wailing mouth. The child begins to feed and yet, at first, still cries until the satisfying milk reaches and appeases the hungry stomach. Only then does the child settle down and peacefully finish the feeding. The inner satisfaction of the warm milk now generates a perception in the infant that the whole world is safe and peaceful. The child's eyes close, the body relaxes and sleep comes easily.

As adults, we develop an accurate perception of *what is me* and *what is not me*, but the stability of this perception only exists when we are not under undue stress. Ask the boss' secretary under what circumstances she avoids her boss and she'll say, "When he's had too busy a day to eat," or, "When he's hung over," or, "Just after his wife calls him for the third time in two hours." His secretary knows that her boss, under stress, may not be able to discriminate between his hunger, his hangover, his wife's harrassment, and her secretarial performance and so she avoids getting caught in his angry, painful, unbounded world.

If we are to function in life with a minimum of stress, we must learn to avoid doing what this secretary's boss does — we must SHARPEN BOUNDARIES under stress and learn to reestablish inner peace, harmony and discipline. The boss in this case would have been much better off telling his secretary clearly and directly, "Look, I'm having a pretty tough time with this budget. Try to keep all unnecessary calls and hassles away from me and, if you don't mind, could you get a sandwich for me so that I can have a working lunch." At that point, if his secretary permitted unnecessary distractions to penetrate his office, he would be correct to chew her out, defending the integrity of his clearly defined boundaries.

We must learn to define the limits and qualities of our life space and then learn to defend the borders when necessary so that inner peace and harmony can be maintained.

Consider the life space diagram below:

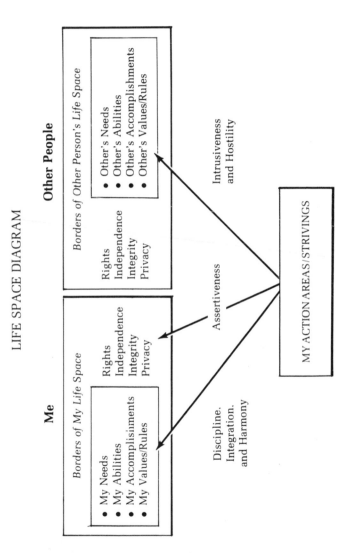

There are three action areas in which a person can operate:

1. *Within the privacy of one's own life space* we are free to recognize and fulfill needs, be proud of our own accomplishments, and live by our own value system and rules. We strive for discipline in our talents and abilities; integration and harmony between needs, abilities, values and accomplishments. Inside this sphere we are completely free and unaccountable to anyone else.

2. *At the borders of one's own life space* we exercise our rights vis-à-vis others; we demonstrate through our actions that we are independent; we have a pride in ourselves that is seen by others as a sense of integrity; and we guard our privacy from the intrusion of others. In this sphere we act assertively in relation to others by declaring and defending, if challenged, our rights, independence, integrity and privacy.

3. *At the borders and within another person's life space* we are an invader and our actions in this sphere are intrusive and hostile. If invited into another person's life space, we are at most a visitor and must act in accordance with that role. We are not responsible for fulfillment of the other person's needs, we don't control their abilities, we are not responsible for their accomplishments or failures, we do not set up rules and establish values for their existence. To attempt to act in this way on behalf of someone else is doomed to failure, as usurping their functions and rights weakens them and doesn't strengthen us.

True and effective assertiveness is only possible when *enacted by a person for himself.* The individual who takes over another person's life, whether by invitation or force, is not assertive, but hostile and destructive. Nature has endowed us all with one additional flaw that undermines our ability to develop ourselves creatively and independently — that is, our *life-long addiction to dependency.* We invite invasion and never fully outgrow the desire to have someone else take over responsibility for our own destiny.

The Dependency Addiction

Our beginnings in this world are in a totally dependent framework. Survival of an infant is only possible if it is able to express and accept its dependent role and if those around it are able to predict, understand and fulfill its needs. From there forward, the developing child faces a series of disappointments with respect to dependency. Mother isn't always on time with the bottle. The child must learn to satisfy itself temporarily with a memory of a previous feeding until the bottle finally arrives. You have noticed with your own children that as they mature, their ability to wait for gratification grows. They cry for a feeding; then they hear mother rattling around the kitchen preparing the bottle and stop crying. Hunger has temporarily been appeased by the knowledge that food is on the way. If the delay is too long, the child begins to cry once more and panic may ensue. If the crying stops this time, it is due to *despair and withdrawal*.

This sequence, unfulfilled need → expectation that someone else will eventually satisfy the need → despair and withdrawal, is not restricted to infancy. Some adults constantly, and all of us under severe stress, go through this cycle in one way or another. The man whose business is in severe financial straits may dream about that "one big deal that will turn things around" rather than clearly confront the difficult day-by-day task of slowly pushing his business forward. When the miracle doesn't happen, he may withdraw his energy rather than renewing his efforts, blaming the failure on others: the union, the bad market for his goods, "bad luck," or his partner for not carrying his share of the load.

The woman whose marriage is failing may let herself go — becoming emotionally sloppy and physically unappealing, blaming the marital difficulties on the "other woman" or her husband's demanding job. Rather than working to rejuvenate herself and invest her energies in redesigning her life and her marriage, she blames others and withdraws in despair.

The student with poor grades has learned to blame the "lousy school," the "boring teacher" or the "irrelevance of the subject" rather than his own laziness or confusion. Rather than spending extra time on his weak subjects, he spends more time on his strong subjects and tries to avoid or drop the weak courses.

In all cases, the infantile sequence of *dependency* → *disappointment* → *withdrawal* prevails and failure is the result.

As adults, we must realize that *we have arrived.* We are as qualified for life as we will ever be and we must rely on ourselves in order to grow and succeed. We must fight the powerful addiction to dependency that is with us from birth. In its place we must rely on assertiveness. The student feeling "dumb" in a subject must learn that this feeling is an important cue. It must be tolerated and must serve to direct his energies *toward* rather than *away from* the course causing him to feel that way. The woman recognizing the rejection of her by her spouse, must look to herself and plan a self-development program to improve her desirability and self-sufficiency. The man recognizing that imminent business failure is at hand must realize that only he can turn things around through his creative and energetic efforts.

The infantile response is to become *dependent* under stress. The adult response is to regard each stress-producing challenge as an *opportunity to grow and develop mastery* over an area of life.

To enact a continuing self-development program in your life you must correct two of nature's mistakes:

> • Under stress you must resist the temptation to confuse your pain with the world around you and *SHARPEN* and *DEFEND* the *BOUNDARIES* of your life space while trying to promote an inner reconciliation of your needs, your abilities, your values and your achievements.
> • Under stress, you must choose *MASTERY* over the life-long natural tendency toward depending on others to solve your problems or blaming others for causing your problems and challenges.

If you give up the reins of your life to another person, remember that his or her existence in your life space is as a "visitor." You may temporarily need a hand or want to catch a free ride on someone else's strength. But if you fail to incorporate the lessons learned from others into your own repertoire of skills, your growth will be stunted rather than promoted by the involvement of "helping people" in your life. In just this way, psychotherapy often damages, rather than fosters, an individual's ability to cope with stress. If the therapist/client relationship leads to a reliance on, rather than a transfer of, coping methods from therapist to client, the therapy will go on forever or until money or patience runs out (whichever comes first).

The Stress Control Formula for Self-Development

The decision to live a life of continuous growth and self-renewal means you will undergo constant change. Since stress is an inevitable accompaniment of change, you will be undertaking a stressful life if you choose to develop to your fullest potential. Proper control of stress in this type of lifestyle is essential for maintaining optimum health and avoiding unnecessary wear and tear on your body, mind or emotions.

Since we know that:

$$\left\{ \text{Your Ability to Cope} \right\} \quad \begin{matrix} \text{Varies} \\ \text{inversely} \\ \text{with} \end{matrix} \quad \left\{ \begin{matrix} \text{The Number and} \\ \text{Complexity of Tasks} \\ \text{Confronting You} \\ \textit{and} \\ \text{The Time Pressure} \\ \text{You Are Under} \end{matrix} \right\}$$

in order to deal effectively with the stresses of self-development you must:

1. *Reduce* the number and complexity of changes you wish to make in your life at any one time. Learn to establish

priorities and set attainable goals. Then implement the desired change in bite sized amounts.

One woman, unhappy with her life at home and feeling chronically anxious and depressed, decided that she should seriously contemplate divorce, should go back to school and change her ways of dealing with her friends from "superficial suburban plastic relationships" to "meaningful adult relationships." She proposed to enact her master plan at once — and so she precipitated a marital crisis, went to war with her friends and enrolled in college. When she first saw me in consultation she complained of acute anxiety attacks and palpitations, the result of stress overload of her mind, emotions and cardiovascular system.

We worked to reduce the number of things she planned to accomplish to just one immediate task. She chose going to school. I convinced her to take only those courses she would enjoy and at which she could succeed rather than to load herself down with courses directed toward her ultimate career path.

She began to find great reward in her achievements at college. Students and her professors respected her and told her so. Her husband boasted about her achievements to his friends. She was delighted to see his respect, admiration and support for her revealed in this way and their relationship improved. She found that when she initiated a "meaningful" conversation with her friends, they were capable of responding. They looked forward to hearing about her new insights in political science and some of them were encouraged to return to college themselves.

Pick one task for self-development and work hard at it until you succeed. Once you get the ball rolling, other beneficial changes will happen with less stress than it took to overcome your initial inertia. Taking a shotgun approach to self-development intensifies stress and defeats your attempts to cope.

2. *Reduce* the self-development time pressures confronting you. While some changes must be made on a timetable (for example, completing a college course), in most cases, change

requires no timetables, or you are in a position to establish your own schedule.

When I wanted to broaden my own life, among other changes I made was my decision to fulfill a childhood dream and learn how to fly. As my friends heard about my new ambition and interest, one of them chided me for taking so long before soloing. "You've got fifteen hours of flying time," said he. "When are you going to solo? Are you chicken or something? I soloed in only six hours. What's wrong with you?" This friend failed to announce to the group, however, that despite beating me by nine hours to solo in an airplane, he never got to finish out the training program and never was granted a pilot's license. I frequently take him for rides in my airplane and give him a turn at the controls in an effort to help him overcome his hidden fear of going all the way through to completion of his training. My generosity came about as a result of his confession to me one day that he panicked during his solo flight and, after landing the plane, never flew again. He had rushed to a goal on a schedule, rather than being guided by his own confidence and skill, and the stress of too much time pressure did him in.

3. *Increase* your ability to cope with change, growth, success and failure. In this regard, there are four major tasks that must be achieved:

- Learning to cope with other people's jealousy and envy, their anger and the possibility that sometimes your gain may be their loss.
- Learning to cope with your own guilt feelings and fears, your greed, your own aggression and your ability to tolerate failure and accept success.
- Learning to express yourself assertively when appropriate.
- Learning how to unload stress and renew your energy for sustained progress in self-development.

Other people's envy and jealousy are endorsements of what you are doing. It indicates that you are becoming someone that they wish they could be.

Other people's anger at you when you sharpen and defend the boundaries of your life space is to be expected, especially if they are accustomed to owning and controlling a part of you or all of you. You need to be clear in explaining to them that by reclaiming your life space you are not rejecting them. Instead, as in the case of one woman, she told her husband, "I want to experience some of the frustrations and also the rewards of building a successful career. Your mastery over your life has been an inspiration to me. Don't let it become a monopoly." If others persist in being angry at you for running your own show, that's their problem and you neither have to live with it nor be accountable to them for actions they claim "makes me angry."

Certainly, by investing more energy in your own growth, you will have to withdraw it from somewhere else. You will put in less time as a mother, a worker, a son or a best friend. Someone will inevitably complain about their loss of your energy. This is a good time to sharpen and defend your boundaries.

"Mommy, why can't you be home when I get back from school," said one child. Rather than reply in an apologetic or guilt-ridden manner, his mother replied, "Because I'm proud of myself and I enjoy my work. When you grow up, I hope you'll find something to work at that you enjoy. In the meantime, Marie can give you your milk and cookies and get you started with your homework."

I'm me and *you're you*, this mother said. She presented her son with a role model of a contented adult, a person he could respect and emulate, rather than trying to cater to his *preference* but not his *need* that she be home to hand out milk and cookies.

Learning to cope with guilt feelings comes naturally after you have reclaimed your right to live within your own life space by your own rules. You have a right to have life pay off for you. If you want to grow, you must evaluate every move you make using the standard "Is this going to help me grow? If not I don't need it."

Minority groups, in their struggles for equality and advancement, have always evaluated all social acts in accordance with "whether the lot of blacks is improved or harmed by this new law," or "whether this new government is good or bad for the Jews." No matter what their differing positions may be on other topics, successful members of minority groups hold formal or informal caucuses to evaluate every decision or event from the standpoint of whether it will help or hurt the cause of their group's advancement in society. Individuals seeking self-renewal and advancement must caucus with themselves, evaluating each decision and event in life from a similar standpoint of personal gain or loss.

Coping with fears is accomplished by saying to yourself, "What would be the worst thing that could happen if this fear was realized?" By doing this you can then lay out and rehearse options for coping with these eventualities should they occur. In most cases, by rationally analyzing them, the fears and their impact on you will diminish and you will be able to live with them while still coping with the challenges that face you.

Greed is not a dirty word. There are only two types of people in the world: those who admit to being greedy, and those who engage in self-deception. If you are an adult, you have the privilege and the responsibility of caring for yourself. One measure of whether or not you are doing that job well is how easily you can name at least one thing you did today from which you alone were the beneficiary. If you can't, you are not greedy enough — or, translated into softer language, you are not taking good enough care of yourself.

Aggression is within all of us. Without it we wouldn't survive one day. Watch an infant suck its bottle — that's aggression. Watch a good student dig into a pile of homework — that's aggression. Make love to your spouse — your aggression is essential to successfully completing that act. The direction and form of your aggression during lovemaking is guided by your sexual sensations. Your sexual urges are powered by aggressive energy. Combined, there is enjoyable sex. Delete aggression, and sexual satisfaction is not possible. Instead, you have either impotence or frigidity.

Learn to distinguish between aggression and hostility, the former being a description of the force which powers all your actions, the latter being a destructive use of that force. To think and act aggressively may feel the same inside as being hostile but it is not the same in results or intent.

Executives who fail at their work do so more because of their inability to accept success than their inability to achieve it. When you win, you carry a burden with you. You are reminded of others who are important to you who have not been as fortunate. The spotlight is on the winner and many people prefer the darkness and anonymity of the also-ran. There is comfort in being part of the crowd of losers. There is a good deal of tension standing alone as a winner. Some people can't carry this load for too long and hence they sabotage their own success. Others, while enjoying success, fear the possibility of failure. "I don't want to fall from such a height. I think I'll climb down to where it's safer in case I fall from success." These sentiments are strong hidden obstacles to success. "I don't want to get too close to you — I'm afraid I'll get hurt," said the fellow to his girl friend. "I'm afraid if I buy a Cadillac, it will get ripped off or dented. Maybe I should buy a less expensive car," said the successful Wall Street broker. "I topped my class at school. Now all the kids call me 'the brain' and they can't wait until I make a mistake so that they can tease me," said the bright student.

If you fear success and failure, remember that you own the abilities that got you to the success you now enjoy. They belong to you forever. If you fail, you will get up off the floor, shake off the dust, and start over again with all your talents intact. Losing one battle doesn't rob you of your abilities to win again.

"Whenever I try to act assertively I never get past the first three letters of that word," is a complaint often expressed to me in different ways by many of my patients. When people try to put their desires for personal growth into action in an effective and competent way they develop a *fear of the extreme.*

Timid people fear that "If I get angry, I might kill someone," and so they retreat to greater timidity. People living a life of extreme self-denial fear that if they begin to indulge themselves, they "won't know where to stop." And so when the need arises to be self-indulgent, assertive or angry, they are awkward, fumble and fail.

What you must realize is that the reason *you fear the extreme is because you are at the opposite extreme.* You have a too great sensitivity to aggression or self-indulgence. You overreact to normal increments of aggression or self-indulgence because to you the "volume is always up too high" for these emotions or traits. You spend your life trying to "turn the volume down on aggression and greed." Instead, if you are too sensitive to aggression or self-indulgence, learn to increase your tolerance rather than trying to get along in life without these essential traits. Learn to modulate your aggression and self-indulgence. Don't just turn them off for fear they will be too powerful.

If you wish to be effective in developing yourself, you must learn to unload stress that builds up in you as you engage in aggressive and challenging behavior. Mental stress can be relieved by learning deep relaxation methods through biofeedback or meditation techniques. Physical stress can be relieved through practicing deep relaxation several times a day, and using partial relaxation methods wherever and whenever possible. While I drive my car or fly my airplane, I consciously take an inventory of my physical status (muscle tension, coldness or warmth of hands, etc.). Then I do simple relaxation exercises which biofeedback training has taught me to accomplish without losing mental alertness for the task being performed.

I constantly live by the philosophy, "Because I have chosen a life of high achievement, that does not mean that I must beat up my body, mind and emotions as a requisite price for success." I off-load tensions at every opportunity and find that the pace of my self-development increases as I dump these unnecessary pressures. In Chapter 12, I will review in detail specific methods for accomplishing the task of controlling stress in your life.

Now That You're the Leader, Make Sure That There Are Some Followers

Those of you who have been successful at gaining power in your home life or in organizational or business life, know the perils and stresses of using this hard-won commodity. Mistrust, suspicion, catching flak from above and below, being revered one moment and vilified the next are only some of the prize experiences that you are handed as a reward for your success. The stresses of getting, wielding, delegating and defending power are heavy and often devastating. You realize that power must be taken, it cannot be given to you. Once taken, it must be defended.

And once possessed, it must be used or it will atrophy. You become the boss because you have the ability to *worry productively*, keeping your finger on the pulse of things constantly, heading off problems and putting out fires all the time. There is no respite for the person who worries productively because you know that it is less stressful to *cope now* than to undo a disaster later.

You also learn that while you can delegate authority, you cannot delegate responsibility. If things go sour, it's your enterprise and you pay the price, no matter whose action caused the problem.

Finally, you realize that only by learning to capture the winds of other people's energies can you sail and steer the ship, so you must learn to support the growth and enthusiasm of your people. What is true for a business also holds true in family life. Only by capturing the imagination of a child's mind can you truly lead and guide. By using repressive tactics, you will retain the mantle of leadership but will have no loyal or enthusiastic followers.

The chief stress points of authority relations between people are as follows:

1. *Trusting* the leader to fairly represent your needs. Trusting your followers to back you in your decisions. This can only be achieved if leadership is constantly reconfirmed through participation of the membership. If not, undermining the leader will become the favorite office pastime.

2. *Communicating* without fear of reprisal. Human organizations are held together and operated solely by communication, not by structure. Let your employees know the problems your firm faces and they will rise to the occasion with greater productivity. Try to squeeze more work out of people through using the power of your office to intimidate them and you will meet passive resistance and sabotage. In a family, these principles hold equally true. Tell the children that you expect more out of them because they are capable of more and you need their help, and they will rise to the high standard of your expectations. Try to force your wishes upon them because "I'm your father and you'd better listen to me," and you will get

surface compliance at best and rebellion, inner or overt, as an accompaniment.

Tell people what they *need to hear*, not what they *want to hear*. The results of the former are short-term irritation and long-term trust. The results of the latter are short-term amiability and long-term loss of credibility.

3. *Remaining task-focused* rather than making decisions that satisfy your ego is one of the best ways of reducing stress in authority relations. Your co-workers, your boss, your subordinates and your family will all be more eager to pitch in and help in a task that provides mutual gain than in tasks that serve to embellish your ego. Forcing or insisting that people honor your position will lead to a desertion of respect. Showing yourself as a capable leader, dedicated to helping get the job done will inspire respect and admiration.

4. *Respecting boundaries* that have been freely erected by people because of their mutual good feelings is a winning way to encourage a dedicated followership. Violating these boundaries or attempting to break up these groups founded on personal friendship and trust, will lead to rebellion and/or desertion. Sometimes a leader must be a "new broom that sweeps clean." Usually, this is a result of the feelings of powerlessness that his followers felt in not participating in the election or selection of the leader. They dig in and blindly rebel in order to feel more powerful and in the process disrupt the organization. Entire departments have been fired or decimated as a result of these types of conflicts.

If a new leader is smart, he will ask for an opportunity to meet with these informal but emotionally powerful groupings before taking office and perhaps even before accepting the job. Making peace and encouraging mutual support with emotionally bonded groups that have predated you is a smart, effective move to make in organizational life.

The key to good authority relations in an organization or in a family is to *avoid feelings of powerlessness in the membership*. If that is achieved, there will be less stress, more work done and more contentment for all members. Leaders lead without undue stress when all members recognize the *advantages to themselves* of effective leadership.

The Mid-Life Awakening

Now you've arrived. You have achieved success. The purpose of your self-development has been realized. You have adapted successfully to changing needs as you grew and matured. Then, suddenly, came a time in life when you said, "Is this all there is — is this what I've been struggling for all these years? Is it never going to get better than this?"

This phase of life has been termed "the mid-life crisis" by many authors. I prefer to label it "the mid-life awakening," because, although it is experienced as a crisis, the urgency and conflict come about as a result of an awakening of the individual to a renewed, intense desire for growth after a period of predictable movement to a life goal. Suddenly, the successful lawyer with a growing practice sees his life as a treadmill and wants to expand his interests, even at the cost of giving up his practice. The woman having successfully raised children to adolescence suddenly is bitten by an intense urge to chuck the marriage and the maternal role and rediscover herself.

The mid-life awakening is a time when suddenly you seem to be able to lift yourself out of the context of your comfortable, predictable and successful life and look for new and greater distances to travel. You can look forward all the way to your own death and become frightened by it. You may feel compelled to increase the stresses on yourself by developing a time urgency to get all your life goals accomplished before your strength and health wane. From the summit of your new awareness, you scan the horizon of your youthful dreams, and with clarity and validity predict which are attainable and which have to be abandoned forever. Long-buried desires are revealed as you scan backwards to your youth. You insist that your opportunities for self-development cannot and will not end here.

This period is highly stressful for individuals passing

through it, as attested to by their high incidence of health problems and disruption in occupational performance and marital life. If successfully navigated, the individual passes out of this phase with a renewed self, a renewed marriage and a renewed dedication to occupational and avocational pursuits. When this phase is poorly handled, the individual may engage in hastily conceived and clumsily executed changes of major import. Sudden divorce, job resignations with little alternative planning, and severe emotional and physical illnesses are the rule rather than the exception in a poorly handled mid-life phase.

The stress control approach is important to keep in mind:

1. *Reduce* the number of changes you wish to attempt at any one time. In the mid-life awakening so many avenues look appealing that you are tempted to go off in all directions at once, intensifying stress and diminishing your ability to cope.

2. *Reduce* time pressure on yourself. You have seen down the road all the way to your own death. Putting time pressure on yourself to accomplish your goals will only hasten the sapping of your energies. If you see an ever-shortening road in front of you, take *more*, rather than less rest stops. Pace yourself to reduce stress and live longer.

3. *Increase* your ability to cope by *focusing* on the key areas of your needs as revealed through your mid-life awakening. Do you want to renew your marriage? Then stick to this task. Changing jobs, or traveling to Europe or buying a new house will do nothing to improve your relationship.

4. *Rehearse* mentally the positive solution to your needs. Don't jump into action and quit your job or sue for divorce. Contemplate all the alternatives before you, and play them out in your mind over and over again. Speak to friends about your plans. Seek someone you respect who has successfully negotiated this stage of life and talk out your plans.

5. *Implement* your top priorities without fear of other people's jealousy, envy, anger or loss. Don't be deterred by

your own fears or guilt feelings, by your discomfort at acting aggressively, or by your fear of failure. Express yourself assertively — don't ever trade away your rights, independence, integrity and the privilege you have to maintain a private life into which no one has a right to intrude. You may have come to this stage of life wrapped up for so long in a marital or occupational skin that you forgot that there is a person living inside. That person has needs, abilities, achievements and values that must be protected, cared for and brought into harmony with each other.

6. *Unload* unnecessary stress through learning to relax and demobilizing any effort the moment it is not needed. Stretching to the limit of your resources when challenged by a problem will result in success only if you have conserved your energies and prevented the unnecessary wear and tear on your mind, body and emotions that stress overload can produce.

Self-development, self-renewal and mastery over challenges are all possible if stress is controlled. Breakdowns in the growth process take place when your ability to control stress fails. You defeat yourself by regressing into infantile blame and dependency rituals which never solve, only delay or prevent, solutions to life challenges. Instead, sharpen your boundaries and become self-reliant when challenged. Your survival depends on you. Maintain your sense of personal responsibility for your life and you will have maximum control in stressful situations.

The species which survive forces that make many other species extinct are always more versatile in adapting to and living in harmony with their environment. Fight your inborn drive to fulfill to a maximum your own potential and you will be at war with your inner environment: your needs, talents, abilities and values. Learn to develop your potential, even though constant self-renewal is required, and you will live in harmony with your inner environment, stress will be minimized and a maximum of well-being will be attained.

6
The Stresses
of Interpersonal Life

Am I Who They Say I Am?

There is perhaps nothing as frustrating as being involved in a conversation or an argument with someone who continually reacts to you as if you were someone you don't know. The policeman who stops you for speeding and talks to you as if you were a reckless adolescent is sure to drive your blood pressure up a few notches. Talking to your bank manager about an overdraft on your bank account can make you feel like an embezzler. Your wife, husband or lover, reacting to your impending trip as if the moment you step on the plane the orgy will start, can make you feel like the cad of all time. Of course, you resist these attributions and insist that you are who you are.

Sometimes, despite the fact that you have always been open and honest in your dealings with people, they misperceive you and their opinion cannot be swayed by your defense of yourself and your obvious irritation. You become involved in a conflict originating in your knowledge about your own makeup and attitudes versus the way you project yourself or are perceived by the other person. "Which *me* is the *real me?*" you may wonder at times. "Am I as indifferent as my wife alleges?" "Am I as naive as my boyfriend claims?" "Are my parents right in arguing that I allow my husband to take advantage of me?"

Confusion reigns at times, with respect to who you are, how you are seen by others and who you would like to be. Relationships with people can be infuriating, chaotic and intimidating unless you have a grip on how to sort out the many me's from the identity pile and attach the correct one to yourself consistently. In your attempt to bring clarity of identity out of the confusion and conflicts of interpersonal life, you will find that the person you really are in a *functional social sense* is actually a product of the properties within you and the role into which you are cast by the people around you. If the group needs a leader and elects you, no matter how reluctant you are to assume this role, they will flatter, cajole, or bribe you into believing that becoming the boss is your duty. When a scapegoat is required, escaping the unanimous nomination when it is offered is only possible if you leave the group. Otherwise you will have to weather the storm of criticism, whether innocent or guilty.

There is no escape sometimes from a role that a group wishes you to occupy. However, it is up to you to decide whether you will *both occupy and fulfill the role expectations* of the group. If you are forcibly shoved into a role, you *occupy it* by dint of the group's decision, but you *fulfill* the role only by your own decision.

"I may as well cheat, since they're always suspecting me anyway," is an example of a role being both occupied and fulfilled as a result of group pressure and the succumbing of the individual to these influences. Living in the crossfire of unwanted and undeserved attributions produces severe stress. To cope with interpersonal tensions, it is crucial to know how to extract yourself from the traps of incorrect roles that you neither desire nor can fulfill.

Need-Fulfilling Roles: How to Define and Maintain Them

In your relationships with other people, there are two main types of transactions:

1. *An emotional transaction,* in which your needs and those of the other person are fulfilled or frustrated.

2. *An administrative transaction,* in which your responsibilities and those of the other person are fulfilled or unmet.

Most relationships have a combination, in different proportions, of each element. You love and adore your children. They satisfy many emotional needs for you. They admire and love you, too. You also have an administrative responsibility for them. You must support them financially and set guidelines for their behavior. They, in turn, are accountable to you as authority or administrator of their lives. Your relationships at work can never be "pure business." Just watch the goings on at lunch, after work or at the annual Christmas party if you doubt that emotional attachments are an important ingredient of a business or administrative relationship.

It is important to know the rules and attitudes that govern both these elements in any relationship. In order to elucidate what type of administrative and emotional role you are in vis-à-vis another person, you must examine your identity from the point of view of:

- The "me" as seen by others
- The ideal "me"
- The "me" I need to be

Consider the case of Bill, a talented architect who was in various forms of psychotherapy for many years due to extreme difficulties in interpersonal relationships. He fought with his partners, was disliked by his employees and had few real friends. He came to the STRESSCONTROL Center as a result of continuing dissatisfaction with his job, now reflected in declining work performance. His partners finally gave him an ultimatum, "Get your problems sorted out, whatever they may be, and start producing again or you'll have to leave the company." Bill came for counseling with the pressure of job jeopardy looming over his head and with a history of minimal progress in previous psychological treatments behind him. In fact, he used his knowledge of the treatment process to undermine counseling, saying, "Look, I know what you're going to tell me. I've had severe conflicts with my father who is now dead and I'm acting them out with everyone else in my life." So adept was he at psychological insight that he anticipated every conventional psychotherapeutic move and neutralized it by a preemptive statement of his own which was accurate but misdirected. He regarded *knowledge about his problems* rather than *action based on his needs* as the goal of therapy.

Using the stress control formula, we shifted strategy on him from what he had been accustomed to. Each session started with an attempt to *focus on* his needs. However far he wished to roam into his past life (now familiar territory to him after so many years of psychotherapy), we continually refocused on current needs. It became clear that as a result of his poor relationship with his father, he both needed and feared intimacy. He craved recognition and approval but was terrified of the risk of disappointment in relationships. He set up situations in which he was guaranteed to be at a distance from people and eventually the depression this produced hampered his life and his job.

Bill spent much of his time struggling to please "others" in his life. The *others* of the present and past (his father and his partners) wanted more performance. He developed an image of himself in relationship to these demands as an *inadequate person*. He tried in vain to counteract this self-image with a mask of *competence, aloofness, and invulnerability*. Inside, however, he was deprived and depressed:

- The *me* he saw reflected in his relationships with others was inadequate.
- The ideal *me* was heroic and invincible.
- The *me* he needed to be was loved, respected and appreciated.

Focusing on the *me* he needed to be, we began to *rehearse* and *implement* ways of achieving this goal. We discussed the types of relationships that he was in and they turned out to have an overdose of the *administrative* component while being anemic in the *emotional* sector. His relationship with his wife revolved around running a "tight ship" at home, giving the kids "good values" and socializing with the "right crowd." Nowhere was any thought given to the quality of their emotional interaction. They didn't know how to play together. They had no concept of how to savor sensations, and so their sexual life became a mechanical act directed towards achieving a goal, orgasm, which was infrequent for his wife and a perfunctory routine for Bill.

Dissecting each of his relationships, we reconstructed most of them to include avenues of emotional exchange in more adequate doses. His partners were surprised when Bill asked to lunch with them and when he began to show interest in their feelings and personal lives. He was looser and more candid with his emotions and this invited a more direct exchange at work with partners as well as subordinates. His work performance improved, but only after he had learned to develop an emotional bond with the important people in his company and in his social life. As he enjoyed relationships more, he received greater support, approval and, finally, admiration of his talents and personality.

In order to succeed in reducing the stresses of his interpersonal life, he had to abandon the identities which were based on the inadequate me generated by his relationship with his father. He had to relinquish his efforts at trying to counteract this inadequate image by taking on a role of "the man of steel" which only increased his stress and reduced his effectiveness. The only workable identity was the me of his needs. Only when he found ways of securing hour-by-hour emotional gratification in relationships could his talents and the administrative part of his work be fully developed and appreciated.

Some tips that will help you define and satisfy your needs in interpersonal relationships are as follows:

> 1. Check your important relationships to see if there is an adequate amount of the emotional component mixed in with the administrative role. If you have insufficient emotional rapport with others, you should seek opportunities for fuller emotional exchange with co-workers, friends and family.

In a marriage you can judge the adequacy of the proportions of administrative vis-à-vis emotional roles by thinking as follows: "If my partner's functions could largely be replaced by a salaried employee or employees, then there is a far too great amount of the administrative role and too little of the emotional role in our relationship. We should strive to do things for each other that can only be done by a spouse. No one but a husband or wife can consistently love the infantile side of me, comfort the scared part, or understand the crazy part of my personality."

> 2. Analyze each relationship you are in from the point of view of who you are trying to please or to whom you are attempting to prove yourself. Are you trying to show your parents, at long last, that you are worthy of their praise or love? If so, you are assuming the wrong identity. Trying to be the ideal me usually is a hectic and stressful chase backward in time in an attempt to remake deficient relationships of your childhood. It's not worth it. Don't do it!

Are you constantly intimidated and swayed by the opinions of others? In this case, your identity is too largely shaped by "the me-as-seen-by-others" type of thinking. Take the internal mirror in your mind and look at it each time you are distressed by someone's opinion of you. Is your own image different than the one reflected in their opinion? If so, reject theirs. You know you best. Educate them about who you really are rather than the reverse.

If you are the person you need to be — the true you — then your identity will be shaped by your major needs in life. You will see yourself as a person capable of intimacy, security, respect, love and effectiveness.

> 3. Analyze each relationship you are in to see if form follows function or vice versa. Are you trying to construct an "ideal relationship on paper" with the hope that the right kinds of feelings will be generated as a consequence? If you are, you are doing things backward and will fail. First, define your essential needs and then try to find and develop a relationship that will conform to them. If you are contemplating marriage, for instance, it is important for your partner to know how to tune in to your unique feelings, fears, and aspirations right now! Don't expect that when you get to know each other better in a few years, she or he will learn how to be your most trusted confidant. Marriage doesn't always promote intimacy. More often it produces alienating

forces such as financial burdens and time pressures. The intimacy, confidence and trust must be there from the start. They cannot be developed through training and experience.

Often, you assume a relationship will be "ideal" because the characteristics of the other person are similar to your mother's or father's personality. "I want a girl, just like the girl, that married dear old Dad," is a tune that ushers in as many marriages as the "Wedding March." There are two flaws here: first, you are probably quite a different person than "dear old Dad," and consequently have different needs and require a different type of mate. Secondly, even if you were Dad's carbon copy, you can't be sure that "your girl" is similar in fundamental ways to "his girl." You know your mother from a child's perspective, not as her husband. You enjoy the benefits of her maternal, but not her wifely instincts and skills. She might be a great mother but a bitch of a wife to live with. The same flaws exist in trying to pick a husband. Don't try to recreate Dad.

Define your own emotional needs from scratch — don't use generations-old blueprints. Then look for someone who seems to instinctively tune in to your needs and who knows how to fill them without much coaching. If you do this, you will prevent much unnecessary stress from arising later on in your married life.

4. Examine periodically each role you occupy to see if you are in it *voluntarily*. If not, try to get out of it or modify it to better suit your needs. In addition to assessing whether you *occupy a role voluntarily*, try to judge whether you are *fulfilling each role to reasonable standards*. If not, modify or vacate the role.

Let's talk about the most difficult subject when it comes to role modification — the parental role. By law, and by emotional and social pressure, we are told that if we have children, we must both *occupy* and *fulfill* the parental role. Nowhere do these strictures placed on parents contemplate the parents' changing needs and abilities throughout life. Some mothers are excellent at caring for dependent infants but inept at dealing with assertive, independence-seeking adolescents. "Where did I go wrong?" moans the parent of the fractious teenager. Nowhere, actually, is the answer. Who says that every person must be competent to handle every phase of the child's developmental cycle? I spend much time with guilt-ridden parents of adolescents trying to help them renegotiate the division of labor between mother and father, always encountering intense resistance to common sense recommendations.

"If your husband is more capable of understanding and accepting the child's strivings, let him take more of a leading role now. You've done a great job raising the children to this point. Now move over and let his skills as a parent be more fully expressed." My recommendation is initially met by shame and depression, "I've failed. What should I do now, go out to work?" The guilt-ridden mother in her despair usually points ashamedly in the right direction. Why not go to work or back to school if you find your maternal juices dried up? A defeated full-time mother is much less healthy to live with than an exuberant and successful part-time student, part-time mother.

If you *occupy* but *don't fulfill* a role, leave it, or modify it to reduce stress on you and improve your effectiveness in that role.

5. When you encounter a role in life that you can fulfill with great personal satisfaction, acquire it like a kleptomaniac. I make it a personal mission to get involved in as many satisfying relationships as I can. I also periodically weed my garden of relationships and roles I no longer can fulfill. If a relationship gives you a kick, it's right for you. No more complex justification for it needs to exist.

6. If you want to eliminate a good deal of stress and confusion in getting along with people, learn to replace the word "but" with the word "and" when you describe someone:

"Harry has a great sense of humor *but* he's a lousy tennis player."

"Shirley is a sensational hostess *but* she's having a lot of problems in her marriage."

Somehow, our minds search for a unitary definition of people, and so if there are several aspects to an individual we introduce "but," and let one quality cancel out another. This leads to confused and stressful relationships.

Can you enjoy Harry's sense of humor even though he plays a sloppy game of tennis? Of course! Harry is both funny *and* poor at tennis. Now you can accept and enjoy his wit *and*, at the same time, accept his inadequacy on the tennis courts. Shirley will always be a great hostess, marital problems or not. She is *both* a good entertainer and a troubled wife. You may wish to join her or enjoy her in her strong role *and* support her in her weak role.

Replacing "but" with "and" in describing people lets you sharpen your definition of the **multiple roles** they occupy. These many roles are *not mutually exclusive*. You selectively interact with a person one way in one role, and another way in another role. By doing a better job of discriminating between and interacting with other people's multiple roles, you will be more effective in all your relationships. You will be able to accept a person's weakness in one area while still appreciating and respecting their strength in another role.

Is It Just Another Fight Or a Marital Crisis?

The most complicated of all relationships in life is, by far, the marital relationship. Nothing teaches a person so much about other human beings as trying to live with another person in this kind of relationship. Nowhere can more be gained or lost, more lessons be learned or energy squandered, than in a marital crisis. No situation in life can turn the stress screws as tightly and painfully as a marital conflict that seems to have no solution. In order to survive a marriage at all, you must learn to navigate the inevitable and repeated crises that marriage generates for all people who occupy its roles.

Few married couples fail to recognize the time in their relationship when the honeymoon is over and they begin to experience more fully and realistically what it means to share one's life with another person. Young marriages are carried over this sometimes jarring transition by the tide of romantic feelings — the wish and determination to get through the rough periods in order to recapture the recently experienced ideal relationship of the honeymoon phase. A quarrel between young lovers more often exhausts itself by melting into extra-torrid lovemaking than by moving to a courtroom battle. The experience of powerful, sustained (and probably idealized) love is so recent that it cushions the conflicts of this end-of-honeymoon phase. Loving memories regenerate loving feelings and relationships.

Older marriages have less comforting recent histories. A quarrel between a more experienced married couple is more apt to be linked in memory to previous quarrels, and the hostile feelings of the couple are amplified by such recollections, as contrasted with the amelioration of hostilities that honeymoon memories produce for the less experienced couple. Still and all, the more experienced couple resolves their dispute by drawing on the resources of their relationship among which are: the not-quite-dead hope that the spouse will finally "change" and live up to expectations; the convenience of their relationship — their dove-tailed friendships, shared activities, mutual interests, and economic links; and the satisfaction they share from their joint commitment to enrich the lives of their children.

There is a time, however, in many marriages when the couple suspects or fears that the relationship is bankrupt or irretrievably damaged as a result of the build-up of hostility over the years. This sense of doom or despair is felt more acutely during flareups of repetitive, old quarrels. An individual, seeing no change in a physically painful state, can be propelled by despair to choose death over unending pain, since well-being as an alternative no longer appears possible. Similarly, there comes a time in a marriage when the memory of joy in the relationship is so distant, and the possibility of its revival seems so improbable, that divorce, or the death of the relationship, appears more reasonable than interminable pain and loneliness.

For some, the resolution of this state is a double life: an emotional divorce from the spouse (preserving the conveniences of marriage and family life), along with a search for emotional union outside the marriage. The "other woman" or "other man" can provide the emotional condiment that makes a dreary but convenient marriage palatable.

The marriage may erupt into a set-piece artillery duel between the spouses where the children may be both the primary casualties and ammunition in the war of attrition. Or guerilla warfare may result, with each spouse lunging at weak spots in the other, believing erroneously that you can kill off the bad and still preserve the good in the population of individuals you wish to dominate and merge with.

Other couples react to the threat of divorce by establishing a pseudo-relationship, wherein the satisfaction derived in outside activities masks the emptiness of the relationship. Frenzied entertaining, dining binges, frequently exchanging automobiles, houses, jobs, all can be attempts by the couple to reach for satisfactions outside their relationship that they cannot generate from within it.

The marriage in crisis goes through a bizarre behavioral zigzag course, its direction determined by the fleeting influences of its component parts. The strong love and hate between the couple push and pull the tiller, causing the marital vessel to lurch and turn so violently that jumping overboard seems more dangerous than it really is, and staying on board becomes intolerably sickening and frightening.

Major battles occur. The spouses may engage in vicious name calling or physical abuse of each other. The direction of their day-to-day lives is impossible to predict or control, walking as they do on the deck of this out-of-control marital ship which sails in the tempest of their dissatisfactions.

Gamely, one or both spouses struggle to reach the bridge and to steer the ship into a calmer sea where it can more easily be handled. It is at this point, the time when one or both spouses is motivated enough to scramble to the helm and take control, that the maximum possibilities for positive change exist. A marital crisis exists at this time and, since "crisis" means "opportunity for change," this is a painful but hopeful period for a married couple. While the motivation for change will rise to a peak during this phase, desire alone, without careful analysis of the marital difficulties, will not succeed in saving the relationship.

The basic elements that go into constructing a relationship in the first place can also be responsible for its demise. These must be analyzed and dealt with if you are to remove unnecessary and destructive stress from a marriage in crisis.

The "I-Hate-What-I-Once-Loved" Paradox

I never fail to be amazed at the regularity with which the following type of dialogue takes place:

Marital Therapist

What's the problem? What do you find wrong in your marriage?

Wife:

He's a soft touch — he's made out of jelly. He can never say no to anyone so everyone takes advantage of him. I can't stand living with a sheep.

Marital Therapist:

Remember back to when you were first attracted to each other. What did you like most in your husband way back then?

Wife:

His kindness. He was good to me. He was more considerate of me than anyone I had ever gone out with, even more kind to me than my own family.

Marital Therapist:

What's your complaint about your wife?

Husband:

She's a bitch on wheels. She never misses an opportunity to get in a little dig. She wants to run the show at all times. She's really hung up on power.

Marital Therapist:

Way back when you were courting, what set her apart from the other women? What attracted you to her?

Husband:

Her strength. I figured she'd take good care of me — run a good home . . . you know what I mean?

In virtually every case of marital crisis I treat, the "I-hate-what-I-once-loved" paradox emerges. When you think about it, it's not a paradox at all. People look for relationships which will fill their needs. If you have difficulty expressing tenderness, you will seek someone who can, and you will value that trait in that person above all others. If you fear wielding power, you will look for someone strong to protect you.

As the years go by, you grow emotionally, and you may not need an emotional spokesman or defender anymore. You resent the monopoly your partner has on a particular part of your emotional life, a monopoly which, by the way, you helped to create. You become irritated that your wife hogs all the power or that your husband's generosity seems to be recognized by relatives while yours is not. One patient of mine put it this way:

> *"All my life, I needed an emotional caddy — I needed some-one to carry my feelings around for me. First, it was my mother — now it's my wife. It got so bad that I really believed that I had no right to feel, that feelings were burdensome or were equivalent to weakness.*
>
> *I dried up inside.*
>
> *When I met this girl, she got my emotional juices flowing again. She was able to read my body language and see how I felt at the core. Then, she insisted that I recognize my emo-tions. She encouraged me to grow not in a demanding, but in an accepting way. I feel through her I was reborn into the human race.*

How the wife failed and the girl friend succeeded was in the way each used her emotional sensitivity. The wife's approach was, "I'm more sensitive; let me handle these feelings." The girl friend's approach was, "I'm more sensitive; let me teach you how to experience emotions again."

If a couple is to grow rather than stagnate over the years, each must gain strength from the other rather than being robbed of the opportunity to grow due to the other person's competence.

Solving the Need/Power Dilemma

It might be worthwhile considering what purposes marriage serves in order to better understand and learn how to repair an ailing relationship.

I divide the needs gratified in a marriage into three categories:

1. Social and intellectual needs
2. Sexual needs
3. Dependency needs

For sure, one of the reasons you married your partner was because you enjoyed her or his company. You may have been excited by personality traits, invigorated by intellectual power or intrigued by the mystery of deep running emotions. The social and intellectual needs you have must surely have been in some way filled by your partner.

Likewise, you must have desired your partner sexually in order to want to commit yourself to one physical sexual relationship for the forseeable future.

In addition, your partner must have shown an ability to create a stable home life with you — one that you could relax in and on which you could depend.

But let's face it. Marriage has a monopoly on only the last area; that is, the sphere of dependency needs. In all honesty, you would have to admit that you have enjoyed other people socially and intellectually at least as much as you have enjoyed your spouse. I'm sure there doesn't exist an honest person who has not thought to himself or herself that somewhere there might be a more exciting sexual partner than the spouse.

The only bond between a man and a woman that is unique to the marital relationship is the dependency bond. Or, more correctly, the interdependency bond. We all need the ability to let our hair down, to be weak, to be sad, to be childish, to be crazy, sometimes, somewhere, with someone. That place is at home, in a marriage, and at a time of stress.

Marital relationships that have been sick for years cease to provide a safe haven for gratifying dependency needs. Your partner has too often attacked you for your weaknesses. You are accustomed to defending yourself against criticism. It's no longer possible to safely expose your needs. Looking for someone to nurse a hurt means making yourself vulnerable, and also it means acknowledging the other person's power to help.

In the context of a sick relationship, each partner is caught in this need/power dilemma. If you wish to satisfy your needs, you must acknowledge and expose yourself to the other person's power. But that is too high a risk to run for someone who is hurt, empty and devoid of hope.

Many marriages hang together on sex and socialization alone. But without interdependence for the satisfaction of childlike or regressive needs, no marriage can be satisfying or stable. In order to convert your relationship to the type which permits each partner's dependency needs to be gratified, you must change from the language of attack and control to the language of emotional need. "You never . . ." must give way to "I need . . ."
"You can't . . ." must be replaced by "Let's try . . ."

An emotional explosion should be harnessed to produce movement. "Since we've paid our dues and suffered through this argument, now let's see what we've learned from it. Do we know each other better as a result?" You must feel that you deserve to have a partner who will accept, understand and cherish the child part of you. Without this foundation of interdependence the marriage will fail.

Signs of a Dying Marriage and How to Apply Revival Skills

Many couples or individuals, otherwise capable of intelligent decision-making, move from marital crisis into divorce based on intuition or an impulsive urge to "get the hell out of this marriage." There is an almost romantic aura in the way some people describe the end of their marriage. "I don't know what it was, but I felt in my gut that it wasn't right for us anymore" is a sentiment which blindly rings down the curtain on many marriages. "I just couldn't fool myself anymore" is the preface to a rationalization for divorce that is often replete with self-deception.

Many people move in and out of marriages on exclusively intuitive bases. However, if the decision in question is the choice of one's career, far more than intuition is used. You wouldn't leave your career as an engineer solely because you felt in your gut it wasn't right for you anymore. Although gut level feelings about careers enter into such decisions, you would weigh and study many avenues of modifying your career before deciding to divorce yourself from it altogether.

Why do people rely so heavily on intuition when it comes to divorce? Partly, I feel, because marital crisis is painful and that pain demands immediate relief, not prolonged reflection. Partly, also, it is because when we assess our track record around intuition in human affairs, we tend to remember all the times it served us well and forget all the times it failed us.

How many people have had this experience? A beloved relative of yours is terminally ill. Each time the telephone rings, you are convinced it is the fateful phone call informing you of the death of your loved one. When the call turns out to be from an insurance salesman, a combination of relief and guilt feelings for having prematurely thought your relative dead drives the incident out of your memory. Finally, when the tragic phone call does come, you attribute great clairvoyant powers to your intuition for having known that that particular phone call was going to announce the death of your loved one. It is understandable that people should want to maintain an illusion that their intuition is powerful. After all, when reason fails and accurate prediction is impossible, what is left for one to deal with anxiety-provoking situations other than intuition?

One final reason for the use of intuition in marital conflict is that in the midst of crisis, especially, and at all other times, generally, it is difficult to sort out and rationally evaluate relationships in which you are subjectively embedded. I'm not sure you can ever be objective about any relationship in which you find yourself, but I do feel that you can find some orienting points in relationships.

Generally, two types of marital death occur as the result of two varieties of relationship problems. A marriage can be *overintegrated* or *underintegrated*. In the case of an underintegrated marriage, the partners are far apart on every issue. They have vastly different perceptions; their life goals are divergent and incompatible; their values are mutually and chronically misperceived and misunderstood. They each experience a sense of profound loneliness because they experience no understanding from the other and can feel no empathy with the spouse. There is, in such marriages, an extreme emotional vacuum into which are sucked the children, a lover, a new sportscar, an excessive amount of food or alcohol and anything that promises to temporarily fill the void. The hollowness may remain, whatever remedies may have been attempted. Usually such marital vacuums result in an implosion, and surrounding family members and friends are sucked in as confidants in a desperate attempt by the couple to fill the void and save the marriage.

Sometimes, a lover fills the void for each or both, and the marriage ends that way. The underintegrated marriage is usually the result of diverging paths of personal growth of each member over the years, to a point where the original attraction between the partners becomes obsolete as new and differing needs, norms and goals evolve for each member. Divorce for such a couple should be an event ushering in new opportunities for each partner to grow further, perhaps in unison with a more compatible mate. Divorce, in this instance, is not an action directed *against* the current spouse, but is a statement *in favor* of the actualization of the self.

The second variety of marital death arises in overintegrated marriages. I sometimes refer to these as "Siamese twin relationships." Here, the marital affinity has been so engulfing that both partners have lost their identities and uncomfortably share one confining identity as a couple. Neither partner can see any action by the other as causally separate from the self. If you tell one member that his or her harshness is one reason for the marital difficulties, the response might be, "That may be true, but my husband is equally guilty." Neither member of this unit can extract him or herself from the relationship to evaluate, reflect on and consolidate a sense of personal identity. Both need to lump the spouse into all personal deliberations to an extreme that permits no separation and analysis of individual needs and strengths. Inevitably, the end of such a marriage is violent, as both partners finally explode from the confinement of their overintegrated relationship, and both experience a transient sense of distintegration as the shared unit of identity is destroyed.

Characteristically, such individuals quickly seek out a partner similar in many ways to their current spouse with whom they can quickly reconstitute a near-replica of the original marital unit. A far better result might be a divorce which is followed by a period of personal growth before remarriage or a prolonged separation with opportunity for the growth of each to allow for the preservation and strengthening of the current marriage.

While implosion and explosion are the respective end stages of underintegrated and overintegrated marriages, a constellation of signs and symptoms heralds the inevitability of such an outcome:

1. Every marriage requires a certain minimum administrative effort to keep the enterprise going while the emotional examinations, adjustments and preparations for change are going on. If neither party expends any efforts to keep the household running at a minimal level (paying bills, etc.), or if one partner launches a financial assult on the family treasury for revenge or diversion from painful emotional reflection, the basic survival of the family can be imperiled. If the parties cannot deviate from the course of administrative marital suicide, it usually indicates a concurrent grave endangerment to the emotional viability of the relationship as well.

2. If an emotional divorce exists, and one or both members is already leading a double life, preserving the convenience of marriage but investing disproportionately great amounts of time in another relationship, the marriage may be beyond repair. This is not to say that infidelity equals marital death. However, the commitment of all or most of one member's emotional resources to an outside relationship in the face of the willingness of the spouse to invest energy in changing the marital relationship for the better, is an indication that the divorce has already happened emotionally for one member. If both members are already heavily investing in outside relationships, it's all over except for the decree.

3. Chronic unyielding warfare, incessant monopolistic needs of one member and unending tears instead of efforts

to change, all signal a poor prognosis for relationships. A partner or a couple who compulsively must engage in combat should move that combat to the courtroom where an end to destructive hostilities can be legislated for the benefit of each member of the family. An individual who feels the need to monopolize the relationship to the point where no space remains for the other member to grow is indicating through that need an inability to engage in the type of partnership that makes for healthy marriages. When tears, confessions of guilt or apologies replace efforts to change the quality of the relationship, and when these reactions seem to become institutionalized as the main elements of dialogue between the couple, they serve to mask an abdication of personal competence without which it is impossible to pull a marriage through crises to continued growth and viability. If you are ill, you want tears from your relatives and efforts at cure by your doctor. In a marital crisis, you are both physician and relative to your ailing marriage.

4. You and your spouse may agree openly to engage in a liberalization of your relationship which can serve to hide its bankruptcy, which both of you fear. If you must develop a "contract" with your spouse in order to authorize you to engage in outside relationships, why not reflect on how much trust is missing between the two of you that engenders your need to negotiate a formal contract in the first place.

5. Feverish attempts to symbolize unity often confirm its opposite. A couple who compulsively rush to buy or sell together, have a baby together, etc. as an effort to repair their marriage usually fail. Babies should be welcomed into marriages that are afloat, rather than being anticipated as buoys which might refloat drowning relationships. A home or car bought or sold together can be an activity that gives the illusion of marital strength, but in the back of it lurks marital disintegration. If bartering is needed to maintain a sense of marital union, it is because there is little or no emotional exchange between the couple.

6. Each spouse needs a degree of solitude in order to

resolve a marital crisis. In this protected mental state, important reflection and redefinition of needs can take place. Vulnerabilities are exposed, a new emotional vocabulary must be learned in order to be able to call for need satisfaction from the spouse, and one must examine ways of gracefully lending strength to one's partner. If one or both members cannot permit such solitude to exist for each, then the mainstay process of marital repair cannot occur. Such marriages will not heal and the agony of the chronic wound will sooner or later propel one or both partners to the divorce courts.

7. When either or both members of a relationship fear instability itself, there is a certainty that change and, therefore, growth will not occur in the relationship. The need of each or both members to maintain control and prevent modification of the union rests on a mistrust of the other member's motives vis-à-vis anticipated change. It also reflects a malignant pessimism about the future of the relationship that usually acts as a self-fulfilling prophecy.

While seven indicators of a dying marriage have been listed, they should be considered in the same manner as a physician evaluating physical signs and symptoms. No competent physician would jump from the symptom of fever to the conclusion of pneumonia. Good diagnostic judgement dictates that the totality of symptoms be considered together. Secondly, the response of symptoms is evaluated in relationship to the remedies applied. Finally, the total diagnostic puzzle is considered and reconsidered after time has elapsed to see if spontaneous remission or relapse have taken place or if new symptoms have emerged. Only after a comprehensive review of all symptoms and signs is made in the contemplative manner outlined above is it possible for the physician to prognosticate wisely.

Extreme care is taken in prognosticating about a sick person's life chances. You ought to exercise equal thoughtfulness in prognosticating the future life or death of your marriage. Even after the wisest physicians have made the most careful predictions about their patients' fatal diseases, history is full of instances where such patients act as pallbearer at their doctors' funerals.

Having diagnosed a dying marriage, it is crucial that you know the skills of reviving a relationship and when and how to apply them.

MARITAL INTENSIVE CARE

The marriage license bureau has got to be the ultimate diploma mill of all time. For five dollars, any two people can purchase legally accepted accreditation as child-rearing experts; acceptance into the status position of "stable adults" (as contrasted with the frivolous image usually accorded to "singles"); and are legally entitled to special tax benefits as an incentive to remain married. Every other diploma I know of requires stringent proof of individual competence by written and oral examination prior to its being granted. Usually, there are professional associations which supervise ongoing competence to make sure you maintain and upgrade the skills and ethical standard that the diploma represents in society.

In the case of marriage, anyone is welcome to join the club. "Produce your five bucks and you get in," says the justice of the peace, for all of us. We exercise as much social control in granting people admission to marriage and child-rearing privileges as we do in regulating entrance to "R" rated movies. If you're old enough and have five dollars, you get in! No wonder marital dissatisfaction is universal and divorce is an epidemic.

In order to cope with a marriage in crisis, you must practice certain skills and hold certain attitudes that are helpful in improving even good marital relationships. Let's run through the list of things you can do to reduce the stress of marital crisis.

The stress control approach can be used with great effectiveness in a marital crisis. You must remember to:

1. *Reduce* the complexity and number of tasks confronting you. In a marital crisis it is necessary to notify those around you, including your children, to make fewer demands on you for the time being. Reserve all of your energies for the stressful process of redesigning yourself and your relationship.

2. *Reduce* the time pressure on yourself and your spouse. One great error that most people make in marital crises is issuing ultimatums to the spouse or themselves to "make a decision soon because I can't stand living this way." The chief source of tension may be the time pressure itself. You must learn to reason with yourself that a marriage that has reached a crossroads with many years of life behind and ahead of it should not be rushed down one or another avenue just because you are impatient or are in pain. If you had a heart attack and were trying to survive, you would welcome the respite and protective care provided in the coronary care unit. You must put your ailing marriage in a time/space splint and give it a chance to heal. Don't crowd yourself or your spouse with demands for decisions or changes right now *or else!* Give yourselves the protection of time and solitude so that your bruised feelings can properly heal.

3. *Increase* your ability to cope by adopting effective stress control strategies. *Focus* on the problems of the marriage by discarding stale perspectives and refreshing your understanding of who you are and what you want out of your relationship. In times of marital crisis, it might be useful to ask these questions and try these remedies:

- Is there too much of an administrative and too little of an emotional relationship between you? Then you need to take time to learn how to play and enjoy each other's company again. Attempt to do less together and enjoy it more, rather than the reverse.
- Are you in a personal growth phase in your life and locked into a too-stable relationship? Then renegotiate your role within the marriage. You will often find your partner more than willing to change or modify roles as well. Ask yourself, "If I was single, what would I be doing now?" Very often you will find that with small adjustments in your relationship, you can achieve these same goals within your marriage. If radical surgery is needed to accommodate your personal aspirations, give your partner first call on the opportunity to join you in

this self-renewal process. Don't automatically assume your spouse wants you to remain the way you are now. After all, why do you think you have been attacked and criticized for so long? Certainly not because your spouse considered you perfect.

- Are you able to be childish and weak in your spouse's company? When with your partner, is your pain and fear recognized and relieved, or exploited? Do you react to your spouse's weaknesses by exploiting them or by helping her or him in the process of gaining new confidence and strength?

- Check the general direction of your life. Do you feel you are headed towards the type of life you need, or do you feel that your life has been hijacked by your spouse and you are now merely providing a convenient vehicle to achieve his or her personal life goals. Remember, a good marriage is a vehicle that gets both people to where they are headed. You must try to steer a course that permits accomplishment of a major proportion of both your lives' goals.

- Ask yourself, "Would I marry my spouse now?" (imagining that you are single and free again to choose). Most people in marital crises are afraid to ask themselves this question because they fear that the inevitable answer would be "No way!" However, once you get past the pain and fear of this initial reaction based on past injuries and arguments, you may be able to assess your partner as a real person and not merely as a ghost adversary of old fights. Can you see ways in which your needs and aspirations can be shared with your spouse? Discuss this together and, to your surprise, there may be more willingness, support and understanding there than you expect.

- Try to justify remaining in your marriage on a week-by-week basis. Contemplating your entire future is too much to deal with in a marital crisis. Think about and discuss what the two of you can do to make *this week* better. Building blocks of one-week size can eventually amount to a renewed relationship. Trying to totally reconstruct your entire future will lead to foolish and unrealistic promises to each other that will fail to materialize rapidly enough to satisfy either of you. "I promise that this will never happen again. I'm really going to become the kind of husband that you've always wanted" is an entirely absurd prediction. You can only realistically say in the midst of a marital crisis, "Let's try to have a better week this week than last." You can get a practical handle on a one-week time span and plan your relationship so that there is enough time for each of you for play, work, intimacy and solitude. Keep your marriage under control during a crisis by narrowing your focus to a manageable time span before making lifelong commitments to stay together or go your separate ways.

4.   *Rehearse* an improvement in your relationship through consistent discussion. In order for a marriage to be revived and redesigned, you must spend time together planning and relearning about each other's needs and aspirations. Set aside a *regular time* each week for such a discussion. Let nothing invade this time, no matter how important it appears to be. To sacrifice this time sanctuary is to lower the priority of saving your marriage. In the course of your discussions with your spouse, try to adopt healthy strategies of interpersonal behavior. You will reduce the stress of your discussions if you:

• Remember that you and your spouse both want to be loved and are able to express loving feelings. However, the *language* of your respective emotional expressions may be different. Your spouse may not recognize your loving gestures because they are in a "foreign language" understood by you alone (and vice versa). Ask each other to describe the ways in which you show your love. Don't insist that your spouse immediately change his or her way of showing affection. When you take a trip to France, if you want to get along well with the natives, you don't arrogantly insist that all the Parisians learn English. Instead, you learn how to get by in French. When you

realize that your wife has been showing you love by
being diligent at housekeeping (something of little value
or meaning to you), don't insist on an immediate change
in her emotional language. Recognize and respect her
form of emotional expression and then, over succeeding
weeks and months, educate her to the emotional
language you best understand. If you prefer shared
enthusiasm about your achievements as a language of her
devotion, take the time to teach her about your world,
your values and your emotional language. Both of you
must be "bilingual" to have a good marriage. You must
be as familiar with your spouse's emotional language as
with your own.

- Remember in a marriage that if one person wins, another
must lose, and when that happens, the relationship
suffers. You are not in a marriage for the purpose of being
made to feel inadequate, destructive, careless or
insensitive. *Neither is your spouse!* The other person, if
made to feel like a "loser," will want to withdraw from
the relationship. Therefore, any discussions you have
must end up with *no winner* and *no loser.* In that way,
the marriage will be the winner and both of you will
profit. The only important goal is to improve the
emotional climate of the relationship, not to establish
either of you as the "boss."

- Always conceptualize your relationship in an *additive*
rather than a *subtractive* frame of reference. If you are
articulate and I am shy, your strength doesn't cancel my
potential. Your skill adds to my life; I can learn from
you how to function better in the sphere of your greatest
attributes. I must not cop out and let your strength make
me grow lazy and *reduce* my abilities to function and to
grow. Teach me how to express myself — don't usurp my
growth opportunities with your superior abilities.

- No discussion should result in one partner handing the
other a burden that is too heavy to carry. It is a grievous
error to initiate a process of marital repair by unloading
confessions of affairs and other indiscretions. If you felt
up to having an affair, it's your weight to carry, not your

spouse's. The marriage in crisis is too fragile to support your guilt feelings. Your spouse may be under too much stress to hear your unnecessary confession. Carry the weight of your actions alone. If and when you and your spouse have achieved renewed strength and stability in your relationship and within yourselves, you can consider whether there is anything to be gained then by your confession.

- When discussing what is causing the problem in your marriage, always take more blame on yourself than what feels comfortable. The natural tendency is to relieve your guilt feelings by blaming your spouse for the marital problems. Reverse your thinking and ask yourself, "If she neglected me, did I do anything to convey my need for her attention?" "If he has been overcritical of me, did I tell him how much his opinion means to me and how sensitive I am to his criticism and praise?"

- Learn about the "blind trust" trap in marital relationships. Many people set themselves up for disappointment by expecting perfect protection, generosity and reliability from the spouse. They react with hurt, shock and indignation when the other person "violates the trust" bestowed on them which, by the way, the spouse never was consulted on about whether he or she wished to accept. My plea to my wife is, "Please, never expect me to be better than average in anything I do. I will be selfish sometimes — so remind me when that happens. I may neglect your needs consistently in favor of mine — I'm only human. Tell me, so that I can readjust my behavior. Don't set me up with blind trust and then knock me down for disappointing you. I insist on being human, not ideal."

- If your discussions get into a negative bargaining theme, cut this off right away. "If you refrain from doing this, I'll stop doing that," means in translation, "Throw away this important piece of yourself, and I will reward you by throwing away an equally vital part of my life." The logical end to negative bargaining is bankruptcy for each of you.

Better than this is positive bargaining in which you say, "I must learn to accept and respect aspects of you that are irritating to me but important to you. You must do the same for me."

- Try to use your discussions to achieve an exploration of each other's life roles. Some men *assist* their wives in exploring their masculine roles. Others see the wife's involvement in such a learning process as a *challenge* and say, "It's none of your business — stay out." Vice versa, a woman must assist her husband in exploring her feminine role instead of feeling challenged, ashamed, and defensive about it. Few men really understand and appreciate the importance to a woman of her friendships and community life. Some women don't understand the incessant ambiguities facing their husbands at work. Some men think their wives have it easy at home. Most women envy their husband's freedom to leave home every day and "talk to other adults." Men usually gravitate to monopolizing the administrative role in a marriage — women move in on and capture the emotional role in the family. Each spouse must teach the other to share both roles and appreciate the difficulties of each.
- Finally, if the discussion ends in a conclusion that you must stay together "for the children's sake," remember that children do better growing up with an example of adult life in which they see grown-ups living a gratifying, joyful and self-respecting existence. They are better exposed to divorce if it is problem-solving for each of you, than to continued marriage, if it is depriving, confining and replete with chronically unsolved problems.

4. Implementing a resolution to your marital crisis is tricky and takes a long time. The greatest trap is to expect too much change too rapidly and too consistently. Set your goals as a couple in the way a good athlete sets his or hers. Batting .300 is damn good — it is winning form. In your marital life, a .300 batting average is also a winning percentage. One good day

out of every three is about as good as most people can get it in conjugal life. If you don't rely on your marriage entirely for your rewards in life, a .300 average will feel like a significant achievement. If you restrict your emotional existence exclusively to your marriage, you will be discouraged two days out of every three and sooner or later will throw in the towel.

When you have successfully navigated a marital crisis and launched yourself and your marriage again on a stable voyage toward your goals in a satisfying lifestyle, you will have mastered the most difficult challenge in the arena of interpersonal relationships. You will have learned how to protect and preserve your own interests and needs in relationships with effectiveness and skill. Your partner must be respected for his or her ability to come out of the crisis intact, improved and self-confident. A defeated spouse is undesirable as a partner. A dignified end to marital crisis sees both partners as victorious in their ability to tune in to another person's inner world and make a vital contribution to someone else's life without sacrificing one's own needs, abilities, accomplishments and values. Marital harmony can exist only if both partners can continue their own adult development with internal peace and with dignity.

7
Seven Keys to Reducing the Stresses of Family Life

The Ubiquitous Family

Everywhere you look you can find the strong imprints of the most powerful social structure in the history of mankind — the family. Search the ends of the earth and to the beginnings of time; both the Bible and Margaret Mead's contemporary writings confirm the pervasiveness and staying power of that institution we know as the family. Look at societies in which conventional family structure has been abolished for several generations and you will find the family concept tenaciously clinging to the minds of children who have never lived in or known a conventional family. The Israeli child raised in a kibbutz has never lived in a family setting. Yet, when given human puppets to play with, he or she will organize them in typical family style: one father, one mother and several children grouped together.

Look at artificially created groups, such as an industrial division, a volunteer organization, a psychotherapy group or any other assemblage of individuals, and you will discover the group members are all searching and manipulating silently to construct a replica of the family they lived in as children (or the family in which they wished they could have lived). The woman who had a neglectful mother and competitive sisters joins a volunteer group in which she vies again with her "sisters" for the attention and approval of the group's leader — the mother surrogate. The man in his job is as frustrated as he ever was in family life as a child when his supervisor chastises him for a mistake. He can't understand why he is treated so callously by his boss who now occupies a fatherly role in his life. He expects, instead, the warmhearted, tender support and understanding previously given by his father.

These cases represent examples of a universal phenomenon — our tendency to transpose into every situation the influences of family life. We recreate, in our relationships, all the roles and expectations that existed around us in childhood. We treat people in our current lives not always in accordance with who and what they are but often as representatives of figures from our past family experiences.

One executive I treated at the STRESSCONTROL Center had consistent difficulties getting along with supervisors during his work history. Roger's family background revealed a deficit in his relationships at home. He idolized his busy and successful father who, in turn, spent little time with him and gave him scant praise. Roger always demanded more time and attention from supervisors than he needed or they could afford to give. He saw their refusal as a repudiation of himself and was constantly annoyed with all his bosses. Clearly, he was reacting to each of them as if they were his father. We counseled Roger that he was "looking for the right thing in the wrong place." If he craved time, attention and love, these commodities were available to him from his wife and family; it wasn't realistic to expect a work supervisor to be as devoted as a "good father."

The search to make up for deficiencies in family life goes on in silent and powerful ways at work as well as in the newly created family we, as adults, have the opportunity of putting together to our own specifications. Because these influences of early family life are inescapable and dominate our subsequent group and parental behavior patterns, it is essential to analyze the ways in which a family functions, the destructive stresses that can arise in family life, and how these stresses can be prevented or ameliorated.

GOOD VALUES AREN'T ENOUGH

We have become an "instant-everything" nation. We look for faddish, simplistic solutions to remedy a host of our life dilemmas. "You have the wrong values" is the current wisdom. "Change your values and everything will turn out all right."

Nonsense!

One of the worst falsehoods ever perpetrated on parents is that if their values were O.K. according to prevailing or ideal standards, and if they enforced or imparted these values within the family system, everything would go well for the children. What an assumption! I probably don't have to extend myself too far to prove to you that some great people have grown up in disturbed and unstable families. And the converse is also true: seriously disturbed individuals have emerged from families that both espouse and live according to the loftiest of value systems. The logic softens when we look at it in another context.

Take a football team, for example. Would you, as coach, be satisfied to say, "Just give me some talented ballplayers, I'll teach them the rules and objectives of the game and we're bound to win." Of course not! You would take the innate potential of the players and knowledge of the right rules as a starting point. From there on in, you would focus on *play execution*. Timing and coordination. Morale. The impromptu response of the players to a changing situation. The interaction of all team members in a concerted fashion on each play is the key to success on the gridiron. No coach would stop at giving the team an outline of the game plan. Every play must be learned to perfection. Football games are experienced on a down-by-down basis by the participants. The game plan (or "value system" in family terms) is an important guide but does not determine the outcome. The *teamwork* exhibited on each down is what makes the game plan come true or not.

Family life is lived play-by-play, down-by-down. You come home from the office after a frustrating day, tired, angry, disgusted and your wife fails to recognize your mood. She tells you that you've been neglecting the maintenance of the septic tank and as a result, the toilets have backed up. A marital explosion occurs. An accumulation of such five or ten-minute vignettes is what defines the relationship between you and your wife. You experience your relationship, at an emotional level, in five to ten-minute segments, as in the brief encounter described above.

You may describe your marriage to others in a different way. "I have a great wife. She really runs a terrific home — takes good care of me and the kids. She's a great organizer — always into community affairs — doing her best to make our town a better place to live." But, in your soul, at the emotional level, your evaluation is different and is often unexpressed or even unrecognized. You experience your wife in terms of her empathy with your moods and emotions. How she responds to your needs and feelings in little ways is what sets the tone for the relationship.

What makes marriage different from any other relationship? The adult, responsible, intellectual part of you can find stimulating and rewarding partners outside the marital relationship. The carefree, fun-loving adolescent part of you can find exciting partners, both male and female, without unique need for a spouse. What is different about marriage is that only in this relationship can you expect your partner to care about and respond to the infantile, scared, hurt, needy, dependent part of you. That's the part of you that, like a child, lives from moment-to-moment. The time sense of the infantile part of you is limited to the here-and-now. The peak joys and deepest frustrations of marriage come from your partner's ability to sense and respond to the infantile side of you. This is not to say that a good marriage can exist solely on a mutuality of infantile needs. To the contrary, the only marriages that survive in viable form are those where both partners share something of each of the adult, adolescent and infantile sides of themselves with the spouse. The main point, however, is that the interaction between husband and wife must include an acceptance by each of the other's infantile needs.

This is what makes family life so damned difficult. At some levels, a family is a collection of competing and interacting infantile needs. In the above vignette, for example, the woman had had her fill of looking after the infantile needs of her children all day. When her husband arrived home, beaten by his work, requiring nurturing, she didn't want to read his facial expression that signaled his need for mothering because she was all "mothered-out." If both partners had learned to express the infantile side of themselves in words, they might have avoided a fight over septic tank maintenance. He would have said, "I'm beat — I really need your help to relax tonight." And she might have responded, "Listen, I've had a horrendous day, too. Why don't we get a sitter, go out to dinner and nurse each other's wounds."

The turning points in football games are well-executed plays. The turning points in marriage and family life are five-minute vignettes where the infantile side of each partner is recognized, cherished and protected.

What's true for good marital interactions, holds true for good parent-child interactions. There is no question but that the problems we have in raising our children arise from what children stir up in the infantile part of ourselves. We are reminded by them of what it was like when we, too, were helpless, frightened, puzzled, curious, dumb, angry, dependent, etc. How our parents responded to these feelings in us as children strongly influences our own capacity to deal with these same emotions as adults.

If your child comes to you in tears and your own experience as a child taught you that sadness equals weakness, you will be apt to suppress the expression of sadness or grief rather than to help the child endure it while exploring the solution to the loss or disappointment that produced the sadness in the first place.

Effective parents learn to identify in themselves the stirrings of infantile fears and needs produced by their children. They will use these occasions as an opportunity to empathize with the child more effectively and to teach the child how to use maturing intellect to solve the problems that have produced the painful feelings.

When emotional crises occur, effective parents can *stop* their activities, *stoop* to the child's emotional level, and help the child *step up* to a more mature level of coping. The catch here is that only when each parent's own infantile needs are being adequately met by the spouse, can the parent respond to the child's needs in a sympathetic and an effective way. When I do family therapy and a parent complains to me that his or her child is "too demanding — asks too much of me all the time and I can't stand it," I immediately suspect that the parent's own infantile needs are not being met by the spouse and that the child's appropriate infantile needs and demands are experienced as irritating because they poke at the parent's emotional bruise.

The moral of the story is that, in order to be an effective parent for your child, your spouse needs to be an effective parent for the child in you and vice versa.

Let's Build a Family from Scratch

The best way to understand how your family functions is to reconstruct the reasons which motivated you to build your family in the first place.

Probably, you were tired of the instability of single life and craved a more *stable relationship*. Having gotten married you both realized, after the carefree honeymoon and young adult phases of your new life together, that you wanted to bring a child or children into the world, to love, shape and mutually enrich with your talents, guidance and hard work. You recalled that in your own family, as a child, there was *security* in the family structure. In hard times, the only reliable people to whom you could turn were family members. If you were less fortunate and had an unstable childhood family experience, you envied your more fortunate friends and vowed to create the "ideal" family for yourself when you grew up. As a child, you were able to try out all your personal skills in the *forgiving climate* of the family before putting yourself to the test in the outside world. You could be angry and competitive without fear of destruction; you could be experimental and imaginative without the fear of humiliation; you could be hurt one moment and loving the next moment with the certainty that you would be understood or, at least, accepted, no matter what mood you were in.

When you were under extreme outside stress, the family became *a sanctuary and place of comfort*. Teasing friends could not invade the privacy of your home. You could practice strategies of retaliation with the help of an understanding father, mother or older brother. Even though you knew you might never strike back at your tormentors, it felt good to know that the family team was on your side in the struggle.

Finally, when it came time to spring permanently into the world of strangers, the family became a place where you could turn for *guidance, praise and support in your efforts at self-development and accomplishment.*

If you grew up in the context of a larger extended family, you learned that it functioned as a tradesman's guild for your mother. She could improve her skills at cooking, sewing, knitting, and childrearing by *apprenticeship* to an older aunt or sister. When she and your father had arguments, your mother could enlist the aid of relatives to *mediate disputes* and *adjudicate the claims* of each spouse.

"Do I deserve a new coat?" she might think. "Of course. All my sisters and cousins get a new coat every three years. My request is fair."

"Husbands have to be talked to with more respect," your aunt told your mother. "Remember what happened to Cousin Rebecca when she fought with Alfred all the time? Do you want that to happen to you?"

The extended family constituted a source of additional pressure on the spouses to continue time-tested and workable patterns of childrearing and family life. The new couple building a family from scratch merely had to "follow-the-leader" — the next of kin — and they were assured of fashioning a family that would work to satisfy basic needs at a rudimentary level.

The couple today, building a family from the ground up, also looks to satisfy needs. These are, as in past generations, requirements for:

- Stable relationships
- Security
- A forgiving climate in which to develop new interpersonal skills
- A sanctuary from excessive stresses of outside life
- Guidance, praise and support for self-development efforts
- An apprenticeship as a parent
- A place in which justice can be sought and obtained

In order to create a family system which operates effectively in providing for these important needs in modern times, you will have to establish your own blueprint or master plan. You probably have no extended family to which you can turn. If you do, you will find their advice obsolete due to the rapid pace of social and cultural change. You must draw up your own design from basic principles rather than relying on the empirical experiences of others to whom you can become apprenticed. In designing a family from the ground up, there are seven basic areas of family functioning which must be included in your blueprint.

The Seven Keys of Family Functioning — How They Can Help You Reduce the Stresses of Family Life

Pretend you are a wealthy, sports-minded individual. You have just been awarded a franchise to develop a new football team. The way in which you might go about constructing an expansion club in football is not too different in principle from the considerations that enter your mind in building a family from scratch.

While you ideally would like to create the best team money can buy, undoubtedly you would have finite resources with which to operate, and would have to analyze your needs and distribute your resources in a balanced and effective way. No use squandering most of your money on two superstars if it means leaving fatal weaknesses in other areas of the line-up. You have to recruit appropriate talents to fill all the roles required by a winning team, from quarterback to equipment manager.

You would then hire a coach who would set forth a master plan for victory. He would have to know the **rules** of football in a detailed formal sense as well as knowing the informal rules of how to mold an "esprit de corps" among the players — from rookie to veteran. He would establish a "game plan" for each individual game as well as team-building strategy for long-run success. All team members, and even the club owners, would have to acknowledge and abide by the rules he set forth.

The coach would then work on formations and special units

that would be key ingredients for success. Passblocker/ quarterback/wide receiver would have to drill together as a unit. Another alliance would have to be formed between the defensive backs so that their work could be synchronized and efficient. A winning football team is constructed out of many such interdependent alliances or sub-units.

The coach would then create a play book with coded communication patterns to assist the team in coordinating their efforts. Each play would need to be rehearsed again and again so that the play execution in a real game would be precise and effective. In this sense, the coach would insist on rigorous and consistent behavioral control on the part of each player. There is little room for individual creativity once the play has been initiated on the field. Prior to that, each player is welcome to add ingenious twists to old plays to add surprise and effectiveness to the offense. But once a play has been selected and initiated, the best results are usually obtained if it is carried through precisely as planned.

Finally, a good coach searches for compatible talents and styles. No use hiring a sensational roll-out quarterback if the rest of your team is stylistically more adept at working with a drop-back passer. The coach must be conscious of meshing playing styles of new team members into the total constellation of existing team styles.

In summary a winning coach would build his team by taking into consideration:

- Resource availability and their most effective distribution
- Fulfilling needed roles
- Establishing workable rules and strategies
- Constructing special alliances or sub-units that perform important team functions
- Developing a communication system to assist coordinated action
- Insisting on consistent behavioral control once a play is underway
- Selecting and meshing playing styles for maximum team effectiveness

Two adults, who wish to construct a well-functioning family, or improve the way in which their existing family operates, must pay attention to these same seven key areas. If only one is neglected, stress may arise in that area to a degree that total family life is disrupted. Just as a football coach will produce a losing team through a single flaw — neglecting player morale while caring for all other components of his team's operation; or by recruiting players who are individual stars but whose styles do not mesh — a family will fail to be a supportive and rewarding environment if even one of these seven key areas is neglected.

REDUCING STRESS BY DISTRIBUTING RESOURCES IN A FAIR AND EFFECTIVE MANNER

The resources contained within a family unit are intangible and tangible and, in both cases, are *finite*. **Energy, time, space, money, empathy** and **attention** are just a few of them. When problems arise in family life, it is wise to take an inventory of the distribution of these resources.

> *"Peter keeps acting impossibly," said his mother. "He must be hyperactive, or something. The child never stops doing disruptive and annoying pranks."*

> *"How much time do you and your husband allocate to Peter alone?" I asked.*

> *"Let's see — we go on rides together as a family. We have family dinners together every evening. We're always doing things as a group on the weekends," she replied.*

> *"But how much time does Peter get for himself — take yesterday and let's count up the minutes you and he conversed together, alone," I insisted.*

> *"When I look at it that way, the answer is 'never.' Or, actually, Peter and I are alone only when he's a brat and I have to discipline him," his mother replied.*

Peter knew through experience that the only way in which he could shift the time and attention resources his way was by "being impossible." When mother and father began to give him a guaranteed twenty minutes at bedtime each and every night, his misbehavior stopped.

> "Julie beats up on her kid sister something fierce," said a distraught mother. "These teenage years are hell. I swear, I feel like putting her in a boarding school so that we can have some peace and quiet around here."
>
> "How much privacy does Julie have in your house?" I asked. I continued, "She shares a bedroom with Kathy; the den and basement are communal spaces. She's a teenager and needs some private space. She's beating up on her sister mostly to drive Kathy out of her private territory."

When the parents converted their basement to a bedroom/den combination for Julie, the bickering subsided. In fact, Julie took pride in inviting Kathy downstaris to see her newest poster of rock groups.

Proper allocation of resources is important in order to satisfy the needs of all family members. If you deprive Peter of time and attention, he will deprive you of energy. If you deprive Julie of space, she will see to it Kathy receives no empathy and support from her. Everyone is under increased stress when one family member suffers from a shortage of a crucial family resource.

REDUCING STRESS BY ESTABLISHING AND FULFILLING NEEDED FAMILY ROLES — VACATING DESTRUCTIVE ROLES

Every family needs to have its emotional and administrative roles fulfilled. Bills must be paid; dishes must be washed; troubles must be given loving care and understanding; children must be taught good morals and values. Roles to fill these needs evolve within each family's structure. It is important for parents to see that all family members (including themselves) share in the emotional life and work tasks of the family unit. Everyone must have, as well, at least one family confidant. Each family member must be recognized as contributing something important to family life and, if not, such a role must be devised for that person.

During the course of family growth, some members of the family take on roles which lead to conflict between them and other family members, or which lead to conflicts within themselves.

Two parents may compete for the role of "confidant" to their first teenager. They may push and pull the child so much with their overpowering and invasive "interest" that the child might withdraw in an effort to escape from the stresses of family life.

A child may be both sensitive and articulate. The other children, sensing this, let that child take on the role of "emotional spokesman" because they know he will consistently express feelings and objections for all of them. Naturally, this child becomes the focal point of family conflict as the other children benefit when the spokesman wins his point with the parents; when the spokesman loses, they join in the criticism of him, escaping responsibility for holding and advocating identical views.

"You are both hypocrites," said Pamela to her parents. "You drink like fish. I know you both use pot. And yet you run an inquisition when I come home from a party, smelling my breath to see if there is any trace of liquor on me."

"O.K., if that's how you feel, you're not getting the car any more. I'm not going to see you go out and get killed by drunken driving," said her father.

"That's damn unfair — I never get smashed when I have the car," she insisted.

"Hey, Pam," her brother interjected, "remember the time you were in Billy's car and you both got pulled in because he ran a red light."

At that point, Pam's driving privileges were suspended, giving her brother freer access to the family car which he used as a convenient and safe place in which to smoke marijuana with his friends.

"We're taking away Pamela's driving privileges as an example to all of you," proclaimed her father.

The child who was more honest tried to maintain a more authentic relationship with her parents. Because she was more articulate, she was more likely to defend her rights openly. The "scapegoat" role was assigned to her because she kept a high profile.

The other children gladly let the "scapegoat" take the heat and even assisted in cornering their honest but unfortunate sibling into the scapegoat role.

A stable and effective family is one in which each person's role is determined only by their needs, their demonstrated abilities and the needs of the family. Duties and privileges should be assigned according to the age-appropriate needs of the child, the fairly assessed demonstrations of the child's abilities to perform tasks, and express emotion and the needs of the family at that time.

Pamela should have been allowed driving privileges based on the following:

1. Her clean past driving record
2. The fact that a teen-ager needs "wheels" to socialize in a suburb
3. Her honesty in expressing her emotions
4. The fact that the car was available for her use

Many roles are replete with conflict and difficult to change. Bernard was a timid child due to the sheltering he received when he suffered rheumatic fever at ten years of age. He became a mama's boy in everyone's eyes, including his own. He functioned poorly with friends and in school. Most mornings he got up complaining of some physical ache or pain which almost automatically drew an exemption from school that day from his panicky mother. Finally, he stopped going to school altogether. The guidance officer investigated the situation and determined that the family needed psychiatric care.

When I saw the family in my office it became clear what was going on. Bernard's two younger brothers were quite normal and independent. They had escaped being overprotected since all of mother's attention was directed towards Bernard. The two brothers took care of each other and themselves in a contented alliance. Father was locked out of Bernard's life and also out of his marriage as Bernard's care, by tradition, was largely the mother's responsibility. Consequently, mother and her "sickly" son were free to unite in their respective nurse–patient roles.

In order to repair the damage this was doing to Bernard's development and to the marriage, I had to evict both Bernard and his mother from their destructive roles. People don't easily leave secure roles, even if they are destructive. Other family members don't readily let them out of the cage in which the role places them. The brothers were content to interact and didn't want Bernard "butting in." Father had learned to occupy his life in other ways and wasn't ready to change his ways radically and resume his long-forgotten emotional relationship with his wife.

In society, we assist the process of radical role change by elaborate ceremonies. "You are now *husband* and *wife*," says the minister after a formal and intricate ceremony witnessed by all the significant people in the couple's life. The weight of the minister's religious office combined with the ceremony he conducts help to enact a major role change for the couple. Both their mothers weep but they relinquish their "children" to become "husband" and "wife."

In disturbed family systems, there is no analogous ceremony to assist a role-changing requirement. To substitute for this, I always use the tactic of *verbally labelling the abnormal roles,* that is calling attention to them as "sick" roles. I consistently referred to the mother as "Bernard's nurse," and reminded her, even badgered her, into being aware of how much she was neglecting her wifely and appropriate motherly duties. So uncomfortable did she become at being called "Bernard's nurse," that she shrieked a denial at me. At that point her husband and other sons confirmed my opinion of her role. "What do you want me to do," she moaned, "he's a sick boy." At that point, Bernard's father got angry and burst forth with accumulated complaints. "You haven't been a wife for years or a mother to your other two sons. You've almost ruined Bernie in the process of 'caring' for him."

From that point on, we were able to work more effectively to help Bernard assume the more rewarding roles of scholar, son, brother and friend. He relinquished the role of "sick child" in order to complete his development and his "nurse" resumed her role as wife and mother.

In a family system, all essential and productive roles must be filled — all destructive roles must be vacated, if you are to avoid long-term stress.

REDUCING STRESS THROUGH MAKING FAMILY RULES PUBLIC

More stress is produced in family life through the existence of powerful but covert rules than by any other means I know.

Johnny was a child with a learning disability. His parents had been concerned about his academic problem and his chances for a successful future for years. They were so tense about all of this that the subject could never be raised at home by the other children or even by Johnny himself.

"Mom, I'm having some trouble with this math. Do you think you could work with me?" Johnny asked.

"Sure," said his mother, picking herself up from her daughter's side, right in the middle of helping her with her spelling.

"That's no fair, Mom. Johnny always comes first," said Ellen.

"Be quiet — do you want to be punished?" the mother rebuked her daughter sharply.

Johnny came back instantly with a rejection of his mother's help. "Come to think of it, I know the math problem now. Anyway, I think I'll go over it with my teacher tomorrow."

Two silent rules existed in this family:

1. We must neither acknowledge Johnny's problem nor the special help we give him as a result.

2. We are not permitted to mention the existence of the first rule.

The second rule covered the first. The first rule buried the problem. Everyone was placed under undue stress and nobody coped or profited.

The solution for this family was the same solution that makes some societies just. Rules that govern behavior must be public in order to be equally understood by all and justly applied.

Mother should have simply explained Johnny's needs rather than hidden them with the first rule: "Johnny has a learning problem. Naturally, he needs more help than you do, Ellen. Let me take a few moments to get him started on his math, then I'll get back to you. I know you're upset when he gets special treatment like this, but if and when you have a special need, I'll be behind you one hundred percent, too."

At least in this case, Ellen could have consoled herself with the promise of her mother's support and would have been relieved by her mother's candor.

Johnny would have been less uncomfortable accepting the assistance. Mother would have been able to relieve her conscience rather than try to camouflage the "unfair treatment."

In a well-functioning family, all operating rules must be exposed, justified, and fairly applied. The comfort this provides to individuals can be compared to the difference in peace of mind between citizens of an open democracy and those of a secretive totalitarian regime.

REDUCING STRESS BY SHAPING WORKING ALLIANCES AND ELIMINATING DISRUPTIVE FAMILY UNITS

In the example given where there was a mother-son/nurse-patient alliance, it was clear how the units of family functioning were organized for the minimum well-being of all members:

Family Sub-Units	Results
Mother/Son Nurse/Patient ⟶	1. Bernard refused to go to school.

Family Sub-Units	Results
	2. Bernard developed a feeble, inadequate self-image.
	3. Mother ceased to enjoy her marriage. Instead, she constantly worried about her son's health.
Brother/Brother ⟶	1. While the two brothers took adequate care of their emotional needs, they were denied needed maternal love and guidance.
	2. Both brothers lost their respect for Bernard.
Father by himself ⟶	1. Bernard was denied access to his father by his overprotective mother, leading to a deficit in needed paternal influence and guidance.
	2. Father quit the marriage emotionally through despair and frustration. Instead he got involved in his business as a compensation.

In order to improve this family's functioning, I had to reconstitute the alliances or sub-units as follows:

Family Sub-Units	Results
Mother/Father ⟶	1. Resumption of normal married life.
	2. Reduction of fear, stress, and frustration.
Three Brothers ⟶	1. Improved morale for all.
	2. Improved self-image for Bernard.

In a family, you must describe all the sub-units that exist in a functional emotional sense. Who really talks to whom? Who is whose *real* ally? What effect do these alliances have on each family member? You must reshape the family alliances to return normal roles and growth opportunities to all members. Doing this will reduce both short- and long-term stress.

CLEAR COMMUNICATION PATTERNS AS A MEANS OF REDUCING STRESS

In Chapter 4, we discussed various forms of distorted communications and how these garbled, coded messages lead to exceptional amounts of stress. When emotions are camouflaged, needs remain unfulfilled, and solutions cannot be found to the problems that are silently and painfully generating the emotions. You look helplessly on as someone you love suffers a depression. The stress on both of you is intense. He can't express his needs, you can't read his mind. Both of you suffer.

You fall victim to an unprovoked attack by your wife. You know she's unhappy, but you can't get through her barrage of blame and accusations to lend a helping hand.

Remember the stress control formula for solving problems based on inadequate emotional communication:

1. Deal with emotions when you first feel them. Don't let them build to overwhelming proportions.
2. *Focus* on the root cause of the emotion. *Rehearse* positive solutions to the needs generating the feelings through discussion and/or reflection. *Implement* the solution in a practical and self-gratifying way.
3. Convert *masked* messages into *clear* ones. Express emotions directly to the person intended and not to a *safe alternate*. *Verbally* express all *nonverbal* messages directed at you. And then respond to them verbally, directly and clearly.

No one in the family profits by being spared the opportunity to share a family member's painful emotions. What is a better classroom for achieving skill in dealing with stressful emotions than the privacy of a loving, helpful and understanding family? Being given the opportunity to share an emotion with a family member is a privilege. Rarely will you be disappointed by the response.

STRESS IS REDUCED IN FAMILY LIFE WHEN THE RESPONSES TO GIVEN BEHAVIORS ARE CONSISTENT

Recalling our football team analogy, what would happen if, on each play, the individual athletes decided at random how to respond, at what pace, and in what direction? Chaos would ensue.

Similarly, in family life, if a given event calls forth one response one day and another the next, chaos does ensue.

I am not advocating here a militaristic approach to family life. If you choose to be ultra-flexible, then be so *consistently*. If you like to run a tight ship then do so with regularity. The most destructive forces in family life are chaos and unpredictability — just as these forces undermine the order of a society.

Your children will adjust to whatever dose of freedom you feel comfortable giving them (within a range appropriate to their needs). What they cannot adapt to is constant shifts in your strategy. You cannot ask a child to stabilize his or her behavior when your mode of parental operation is in constant flux.

If you make rules, enforce them — or else, don't bother making them.

If you make promises, keep them. Don't ask a child to respect you through angry and disappointed eyes.

If you require a set of principles be upheld, adhere to them yourself.

Your children will assess you in two ways:

1. They will listen to what you say — this communicates your values and attitudes to them.
2. They will monitor and evaluate your way of life. This imparts credibility to your words. If you are inconsistent, you will lose your credibility and while they may understand, they will not adopt your attitudes and values.

SYNCHRONIZED PERSONALITY STYLES REDUCE FAMILY STRESS

Why do we, as adults, still stubbornly retain the childhood notion that "parents must be perfect?" Intellectually we know better than that. Yet, emotionally, we feel we must be all things to our children in order to be worth anything at all.

All of us have areas of great competence as well as major weaknesses. This holds true in the realm of our personality structure. Fortunately, we can adjust what we do in life to expose ourselves to situations which rely on our strengths rather than jeopardizing ourselves by depending on our weaknesses. This can work for us in all life experiences but one — parenthood. As a parent, you are forced to relive your entire life cycle through your union with a growing child. Those aspects of your own development that caused serious problems for you will come up again with each child you raise to maturity. Consequently, you will recapitulate your own unresolved stressful experiences through your children's growth stages and will be less competent to cope with certain stages than with others.

Judy was highly organized, neat and punctual. Her childhood was similarly rigid and also sterile, as her mother and father practiced suppression of all feelings and elimination of all complaints and protests from their lives. "Keep your chin up. Keep a stiff upper lip," was their motto. "A place for everything and everything in its place," was their prideful saying. Judy's childhood was filled with activity but no joy. She was given values but no love and warmth. She learned to cope with people by being "correct" in everything she did and said.

When she and Jim had their first child, her careful plan for maternal life quickly came apart. The child would simply not conform to her blueprint for his behavior. He was an energetic and curious lad who was all over everything, constantly taking things apart and attempting to reassemble them. The more Judy insisted that he put things away, the more upset they both got. Because the child rebelled, she scolded him. He cried and had tantrums, and she was even more upset at the emotional mess this created.

When I saw Jim and Judy in my office, she was beside herself with feelings of frustration and failure.

"Why do you think you have failed?" I asked.

"Because I just can't handle the child," she replied.

"We both know you well enough to have predicted that you'd have trouble dealing with a messy, curious, disorganized toddler. Your life as a child was very different in style and substance. At no time did you have the opportunity to learn how to cope with messes, either emotional or material. Jim, on the other hand has a looser style. His upbringing was more freewheeling. Your styles of coping are complementary and together are sufficient to raise a healthy child. Let Jim handle the messiest situations. You can learn from him how to cope with your baby's untidy and unpredictable emotional reactions," I encouraged her.

Learning to use different personality styles in a complementary rather than a competitive or mutually neutralizing way is an important key to reducing stress in family life.

To be a successful parent in a contented, growing family, you must learn to size up all seven key areas of family functioning and make all necessary and appropriate adjustments. Good football teams don't just happen because you throw talented players together and dress them in the same uniforms. It takes planning, practice and lots of postgame analysis and readjustments. Good families don't just happen when you take well-intentioned people, cloak them in one surname, and house and feed them adequately. It takes study and analysis, lots of practice, and a diligent review of mistakes as well as methods of readjustment and repair.

8
The Stresses of Competitive Sports and How to Defeat Them

My Skiing Trip to Killington or What My Broken Rib Can Teach You about Stress

This story is true, embarrassing and painful. It concerns a trip I made to Killington, Vermont, with my fifteen-year-old son and his friend to enjoy a weekend of skiing. The net result of the trip for me was a cracked rib and a lot of firsthand knowledge about how stress can defeat you in sports. I'm telling my story here, in spite of the fact that I will come out looking foolish and clumsy, because it can teach you about *what not to do* in sports if you want to remain healthy.

Last November, I arranged to take my teenage son and his friend on a ski trip. I flew into the New Haven, Connecticut, airport to pick them up in my plane on a blustery, cloudy day and loaded the skiing paraphernalia on board the plane. We checked weather at our destination, Rutland, Vermont, and found out that it would be instrument conditions only for landing there. Supremely confident of my instrument-flying capabilities, and my tough and well-equipped Beechcraft Bonanza airplane, we pointed the nose of the plane skyward and headed north for a weekend of early winter skiing.

Arriving in the vicinity of Rutland airport, we were flying totally blind, embedded in a thick cloud bank. We were cleared for an instrument approach to the airport by the Boston air traffic controller. As I initiated the instrument approach, I noticed a serious malfunction in a piece of electronic equipment which was essential for a safe instrument landing. Glancing quickly at the instrument chart that guides pilots to safe landings in instrument conditions, I noticed a warning: "Rutland airport is surrounded by mountainous terrain in *all four* quadrants." "No time to panic," said my disciplined pilot's mind. "I've been through emergency routines a hundred times during and after my training and I will figure out a solution." I took calm, relaxed breaths, made a mental note to relax my muscles, and quickly figured out a strategy of how to use standby equipment to substitute for my malfunctioning instrument. I took several cross-fixes on my navigational radios and then proceeded to descend calmly through the clouds on a precise approach to the runway. The years of pilot training, teaching me how to *focus* on the problem at hand without panicking, and the numerous simulated emergency *rehearsals* given me by my instructor paid off. I *implemented* a safe landing in spite of the overwhelming stress of blind flying with an equipment malfunction. "So far so good," I patted myself on the back as we taxied to a halt and disembarked.

We arrived at the hill, clamped on our boots and skis and prepared for an exhilarating first skiing day of the season. "Peter," I called to my son's friend, "You can meet us here at 2 p.m. after your lesson. Jamie and I are going to ski from the top." Peter was a complete beginner and I had arranged for him to take a lesson that day. My son, a ski racer, and I, an expert skier, prepared to warm up on an intermediate grade slope before challenging the steep expert trails.

"Which way down is easiest?" we asked a man at the mountaintop. "Over there," he said, pointing to a trail with his ski pole. My son and I started confidently down that trail and soon were shocked to see an almost vertical drop of several hundred feet in front of us.

"Jamie, I think we took the wrong way down," I said fearfully.

"Guess you're right, Dad," he replied calmly. "Don't worry. We'll take it in little bites and sideslip when it gets too steep." His years of racing experience had programmed strategies into his mind and body enabling him to cope with any difficult skiing situation. "Dad," he said, "when I first started slalom racing, my coach drilled into me that I must take the hill in small sections: pole-by-pole and turn-by-turn. We'll go down with a stop every 50 or 100 feet." My son's racing strategy paid off. We safely and enjoyably made it down the hill and then we went right back up the lift and came down the same trail again, *on purpose* this time.

"So far so good," thought I, as we descended to the base lodge to meet Peter, whose lesson was over by now. I felt good because my son's strategy reconfirmed so many of my ideas about coping with stress. *Reduce* the challenge to small portions; in this case, ski the hill in 50 to 100-foot installments. Don't think of getting all the way down at once. *Reduce* time pressure on you for completing the task. Stop frequently and talk or enjoy the scenery as you rest up to cope with the next challenging strip of ski trail. As we neared the base lodge I was in high spirits, looking forward to a hearty lunch.

"Peter's not where he said he'd meet us," my son reported to me with alarm. "It's 2:20 and he was supposed to be here at 2:00." We checked with the ski-school desk. His lesson had ended at 1:30 as scheduled. With growing concern, we went to the ski patrol infirmary. "No Peter Tomkins has been brought in for treatment of injuries," they reported to us.

We dashed out, clamped on our skis and searched all the beginner trails again and again. Still no sign of Peter. Back we rushed into the ski-patrol headquarters at 4:00 p.m. — the closing time for the hill. They too were alarmed as Peter was neither injured nor anywhere we searched. The ski patrol prepared a search party to sweep all the trails for a teenage boy we feared was lying frozen, perhaps wrapped around a tree or in a gully beside a trail.

"Jamie, let's join the search," I suggested. We rushed outside. I bent down to fasten the runaway strap onto my ski boot and heard a loud *snap* in the left side of my chest. Intense pain immediately radiated from where the snap was felt. I knew I *had broken a rib*.

Peter turned up moments later, happy and apple-cheeked. "I had a great time skiing with this girl I met. Sorry I was late but my watch got wet in a fall and it stopped."

I was in too much pain to throttle him or even rebuke him. I just hobbled away, listing to my left, trying not to breathe too deeply in order to reduce the pain. I had broken a rib by bending over sideways to fasten a strap — something I had done safely 10,000 times before. I could only smile inwardly thinking of the irony of the situation. An emergency instrument landing — *not a scratch!* An unexpected ski run down the side of a breathtakingly steep hill — *no harm done!* Bending over to fasten a ski strap while standing perfectly still at the base lodge — *one painfully broken rib!* Score one for stress!

The time pressure I was under to find Peter, whom I feared was dying of exposure, turned the stress screws tightly on my mind and body. The magnitude of the problems I felt I would have to deal with was vast. "Will the child be alive or dead? Will he need immediate medical care — if so, where could I have him treated? How do I explain all this to his parents?" With all this on my mind, the muscles all over my body and in my chest were as tight as the stress winch could turn them. Bending over with a body made rigid by stress was enough to cause me to break a rib. Sports injuries are definitely stress-related. Nobody will ever convince me otherwise.

The Greatest Adversary You Have in an Athletic Contest Is Yourself

As you contemplate engaging in a competitive sport, no doubt you focus your mind on your adversary. "How good is the other team? How tough a tennis player am I facing? What type of hitter am I pitching to?" You try to size up the skill and style of your opponent in order to develop a winning strategy for yourself. The problem is, that in competitive sports, the greatest adversary you have is on your own team — that opponent is *yourself*. The threat you pose to your own success outweighs by far any opponent's guile and tactics. You can *see* his or her strategies for victory quickly. You can't, as easily, detect in yourself how many ways you can be undermined by stress.

Your *muscles* work in sets of opposing pairs. Your biceps pulls in an opposite direction than your triceps. The muscles in your stomach that pull you to bend forward at the waist are opposed by a set of muscles in your back that pull you erect.

Synchronized muscle activity, essential to good athletic performance, requires that when one muscle pulls your limb or trunk in one direction, the opposing muscle groups must relax to permit smooth movement. If you remember how I broke my rib at Killington Mountain, you won't forget that stress can defeat and injure you in sports. Stress causes a general increase in all muscle tension. It sets all muscle groups at hair-trigger levels of readiness to contract. Consequently, opposing muscle groups end up contracting simultaneously rather than alternately, giving rise to stiff, jerky, uncoordinated movements.

In order to have a coordinated flow of body action for athletic activities, you must be as relaxed as possible. You must carry out each movement in smooth, definite, and sometimes powerful movements. Relaxation and power are not contradictory quantities in sports. They are essential partners because of the way our bodies are constructed. The most powerful golf swing or tennis swing is one in which the muscles essential for the action contract powerfully, while all other muscle groups relax, permitting the power of the swing to be carried through without opposition.

In Chapter 12, we will review some exercises that assist you in keeping your muscles relaxed while you are under stress.

Just as each muscle in your body has a second competing muscle which can defeat the action of the first, your mind is subjected to many competing thoughts and distractions during an athletic event. Your *attention* must be focused on the next action you will take and nothing else. "Keep your eye on the ball," shouts the tennis, golf or baseball instructor. "Keep your knees bent and lean down the hill," says the ski instructor. They implore you to *focus* your attention on one essential action. Your mind wanders. "I wonder if I looked stupid trying to serve the ball. What if I fall and my ski binding releases? Will I be able to put it on again on this steep slope?" Your mind is continually widening its focus to a range of defeating detail while your instructor tries to remind you to reduce the scope of your concern to watching the ball and winning the point.

You can improve the power of your mind to resist distractions by learning the key movements in each sport. In those sports where clubs or rackets are used, the focus should be on the *ball*. Since you must learn to use deftly the racket or club, which are

unnatural extensions of your arms, the most essential consideration is the ball's location. The racket and club head have no sen-
sory apparatuses like your hands. Consequently, you must make
them "feel" by using your eyes to guide them to their target.

Learning to focus your mind can be assisted by meditation
techniques which, in essence, are mind-focusing exercises. In
Chapter 12, we will review the principles of mind-focusing that
you can productively employ in sports activities.

Breathing patterns play a great role in assisting or undermining
your stamina and energy. Some sports such as football, hockey
and baseball require intermittent bursts of energy. Such sports as
track, swimming and skiing rely on sustained levels of activity.

There are two apparatuses that cause you to breathe. Your diaphragm moves out of and into your chest cavity like a piston,
sucking air in and then expelling it. The diaphragm is used exclusively for relaxed breathing. When more air is required during
extra exertion, the rib cage moves out and in like a bellows, sucking additional air into the lungs. Watch a 100-yard dash and you
will see the runners' chests heaving at the end of the race, trying
to catch up on supplying oxygen to the body that has used up
energy "in advance" during the burst of exertion.

Heavy chest breathing is a major drain on your energy supply.
The exertion of maximum breathing efforts can exhaust your energy. Consequently, unless the athletic activity requires it, you
must learn to revert to breathing smoothly and restfully with your
diaphragm and reserve heavy chest breathing for maximum short
bursts of activity. In Chapter 12 we will outline a useful breathing
method you can apply in all types of athletic activities.

Time pressure has an adverse effect on all situations that require
you to cope with stress. In sports, as in other stressful situations,
you must reduce the time pressure on you. The pro always
makes things look easy. He never appears rushed and *he isn't*.
He bounces the ball again and again at the foul line, breathes in a
relaxed and regular way, and then floats the ball into the basket.
The high scoring hockey player skates down the ice in long, ef-
fortless strides, making smooth, elusive and unhurried turns as he
breaks free and scores. The clever football coach knows when to
relieve time pressure on his team by calling a "time-out." The

successful marathon runner doesn't try to lead the pack from the start. He tries to pace himself for endurance and run to his own winning time schedule. To be a successful athlete, you must use time in your own favor. A rushed kick or slapshot will fail. A smooth, unhurried effort will be on time and on target.

Performance criteria have been developed to gauge athletes in all sports. Batting averages, earned run averages, golf handicaps, numbers of rebounds per game, and every other variety of statistic is kept for every sort of sport in existence. The athlete who goes into a game focusing on these statistics will surely perform more poorly than his or her capabilities should permit. The emphasis on performance criteria increases stress to overload levels, decreasing, rather than increasing, the performance of the athlete. To control stress and function efficiently, you must *reduce* the complexity and number of *tasks* confronting you. This means, you must concentrate on precisely what you are doing at the moment. You should not concentrate on your season average, or the number of points you have or haven't scored in this game. Sports success is won on a moment-to-moment basis. Each play is independent of every other. Each swing or stroke is entirely independent of the ones which preceded it and those which follow it. Whether you score this basket has nothing to do with the number you have already scored in this game or season.

A good coach will drill this message into his team. Each person must concentrate on his or her activity on each play. When you miss an easy putt, that doesn't mean you are having a bad day at golf. In fact, the association in your mind between a muffed play, or missed putt, or bad serve, and the conclusion that "this is not my day" can be the *cause* of your defeat. Isolate your game into airtight compartments. Perform each unit of action with maximum skill. Then forget the action that just took place and cope with the one at hand.

Your *attitude about errors* is an essential ingredient of success in sports. A failed play, serve or stroke is useful information to you. It feeds back a message to your body which, if left alone, will automatically record the information and readjust your performance for more success on the next play. If mistakes bother you, you will become irritated with yourself. Your mind will be dis-

tracted by this irritation; your muscles will be more taut than is
efficient for them; and your reflex adjustment on the next play or
stroke will be impaired or will not occur at all. When you make a
poor shot at golf, you will try to "kill the ball" on the next stroke
to make up lost ground to the green. Instead, you will make an
even poorer shot the next time. If you simply used the poor stroke
as information, you would relax and make a reflex correction on
the subsequent shot.

Athletics are a means of programming your muscle groups to
act in harmony with each other. Irritation and self-criticism disrupt harmony. Information your body receives about poor coordination can improve internal harmony and will subsequently lead
to better performance. Use each mistaken move as an opportunity
to improve. Then refocus on the next play and forget the past
ones. Your body will remember to do what it has to for success.

WITH TEAMMATES LIKE THIS, I DON'T NEED ADVERSARIES

In team sports there are four major obstacles to concerted performance:

1. While *individual styles* of play are essential building
blocks for team success, the end product of all team sport is
successful team performance. An athlete's job is to work
his or her style of play into a successful team effort. The
true professional will modify and subordinate his or her
own style to suit the team's objectives. The "showboat" or
"hot dog" will try to use the team as a supporting cast for
his or her own starring efforts. You may have witnessed
many occasions (I know I have) when a new team member
reaches star status just at the same time as an existing star
athlete's performance begins to falter. Very often, the
existing star goes downhill due to an inner resentment to
sharing the limelight with someone else. This irritation at
having a competing star on the team disrupts his internal
harmony, and the established star begins to fail not due to
lack of skill but due to *inability to fit his ego needs into a*

successful team effort. Rather than accommodating his style
to the team's new needs, he tries to impose his style upon
the team. The usual result is a decrease in his
effectiveness or his elimination from the team via a trade.
2. *Envy* is the enemy of team sports. Many athletes are
more preoccupied with competing for recognition with
their teammates than in beating the opponent. Sports
generate this type of envy by their very nature:

"Will I make the team or will he?"
"Will I be on the starting line-up or will she?"
*"Who will be voted most valuable player — me or my
teammate?"*

In North America athletics, we create a fierce intra-team
competition for prominence that produces stress among all
athletes and reduces overall team effectiveness. In my
opinion, a good coach would do well to eliminate all
incentives that produce intra-team rivalry and envy, and
replace these with incentives for team success. This would
promote assistance rather than destructive envy among
team members. While my recommendation is an
unattainable ideal, the opposite extreme is what prevails
today. It is counterproductive and only promotes
unnecessary stress among team athletes.
3. Many athletes are greatly talented individuals but unable
to excel in team sports due to a fear of *intimacy.* The
concept of intimacy may seem alien and effeminate in the
athletic world. But how else would you describe the type of
relationships that evolve when a group of people eat, sleep,
live, travel, work, think and act as one person for months
on end? Some athletes have personalities that make it
difficult for them to handle that amount of closeness with
other individuals. They throw up walls to maintain a sense
of needed privacy and, in the context of team life, this is
seen as a rejection by them of their teammates. They may be
resented for remaining distant and tensions will arise
between themselves and their teammates.

If you find, as an athlete and/or coach, a member of your team needs privacy off the field, let it be. He or she is only seeking a comfortable existence for his or her personal needs. As long as that athlete works as an intimate teammate on the field, the need for distance from others off the field should be respected.

4. *Communication* among team members is an essential part of successful team performance. There must be communication between team members at several levels:

   a. Formal communication is a part of all team sports. Signals are called — all team members must be familiar with them and respond to them with speed and precision.
   b. Communication must exist between teammates with respect to the quality of their on-the-field performance. Athletes should be encouraged to supervise each others' performances. Peer review of any activity enhances group performance. You must remember that a review of your teammate's performance should include commendation and reinforcement as well as constructive criticism. Many coaches and athletes believe in purely vertical review — coach-to-player, veteran-to-rookie. Group review of every team member's performance helps all the participants be aware of their teammates' style, strength and weaknesses. They can make better group and individual adjustments to each teammate's style and abilities if every player is regularly required to assess the performance of all other team members.
   c. Communication at an emotional level must be encouraged and permitted off the field. Gripes between team members should be openly aired and dealt with as they arise. No athlete should be required to carry the dual burden in a game of individual effort plus the effort required to suppress anger or resentment at a team member.

I'M FACE-TO-FACE WITH MY OPPONENT AND
I'M AFRAID TO PULL THE TRIGGER

Any competitive game is based on the use of aggression to overcome an adversary. Some people, based on their experiences in life or their personalities, experience difficulty accepting and using aggression within themselves. They may have once been violent with someone and accidently caused them harm. The residual guilt feelings may surface each time they call forth their aggression. The dampening effect of guilt feelings inhibits aggressive effort and impedes performance.

Vince Lombardi's famous statement, "Winning isn't everything — it's the only thing," expresses the extreme of athletic aggressiveness. His comfort with being supremely and single-mindedly victorious accounted for the success of his teams over the years. As an athlete, you must learn to liberate your aggression from the bonds of guilt feelings. Drub your opponents! Smash your adversaries! Beat the pants off your competition! Cream the bastards!

The greatest and safest forum for learning to use aggression properly is athletics. You learn to channel enormous amounts of energy into physical coordination and away from hostility. You realize that hating your opponent won't win the game for you unless you divert energy from the hatred reservoir into faster running, more clever strategies, more coordinated team effort and an ability to be cool and relaxed while under stress. The successful athlete realizes that winning is a high and losing is a lesson serving as a springboard for change, skill development, and renewed effort.

To be a truly successful competitor, you must learn to control the stresses that arise from within you; you must fuse your skills with your teammates'; and you must learn to cast off guilt feelings and enjoy winning.

9
Stress in
Childbirth

Lamaze for Mom

We know stress is produced in people who undergo rapid and major change. A person under excessive stress functions less effectively emotionally and physically, is more tense in all respects and feels pain more acutely. What situation in life is capable of producing more change, and hence more stress, then pregnancy and childbirth? Nothing remains the same after the experience as it was before. Your body changes drastically. Your emotions are more labile. Your lifestyle undergoes a radical alteration. And your relationship with your husband must now be modified to make room for the entirely new and demanding role of "mother." No woman going through pregnancy and childbirth can escape undergoing an enormous amount of stress. The only effective thing to do is to learn to accept that fact and cope with the stresses of the situation as well as you can.

A major breakthrough occurred in the experience of pregnancy and childbirth with the advent of "natural childbirth," or the "Lamaze Method." This technique is an excellent example of the best stress control principles you can adopt since it teaches you how to *focus* on important functions; you learn how to *rehearse* effective ways to cope with the childbirth process; and you can then *translate* these preparations into an enriching, stress-controlled childbirth experience.

The basis of this method is learning to relax all functions in the body, thus conserving energy which is then usefully applied to the central process — expelling the child from the womb.

A tense pelvis holds the baby back, making childbirth more difficult for infant and mother alike.

Tense muscles and labored breathing exhaust the mother and result in a desultory labor that can harm both mother and child. A woman in hysterics due to her pain will, through the unnecessary stress of her panic, only intensify the pain she experiences.

The Lamaze technique teaches mothers to *focus* on relaxing every muscle group in the body. Relaxed diaphragmatic breathing is taught and *rehearsed* in conjunction with muscular relaxation. The woman practices these relaxation methods to a point of proficiency so that even the most trying labor will not distract her from the task of controlling her breathing and muscle relaxation — thus controlling her stress.

Finally, during the childbirth process itself, she *implements* these methods and is pleased to find the labor pains bearable. She feels in complete control, having rehearsed her role in the labor room many times over. She becomes engrossed in conserving energy between contractions and focusing her energy during contractions on muscular efforts that help expel the infant from the uterus, while simultaneously relaxing those muscle groups that, if tense, might slow this process. Finally, when the child is born, the mother is awake, energetic and can participate consciously in a miracle of life rather than being gassed, unconscious and exhausted. She ends up healthier and more contented. The infant is born with no potentially harmful anaesthetic substances in its bloodstream. Controlling stress is the magic key to producing all these benefits to both mother and infant.

Leboyer for Baby

Dr. Frederick Leboyer*, a French obstetrician, has claimed that a special technique for delivering babies produces healthier and happier babies at the time of their birth and that this has beneficial consequences for them in later life as well.

*Frederick Leboyer, Birth Without Violence. (New York: Alfred A. Knopf, 1976).

He postulates that the infant is exposed to violence in childbirth due to the stressful, rapid and major changes to which it is subjected. From a warm, weightless, fluid confinement, the infant is suddenly thrust into a cold, noisy world with glaring lights and with the lead weights of gravity attached to its feeble spine, limbs and bobbing head. The infant cries out in panic and protest at this insult to its harmonious state, but we don't listen or respond.

Dr. Leboyer advocates that we *reduce* the amount of change to which the infant is exposed and also *reduce* the time pressure of that change. In Leboyer's method, the infant is slowly exposed to the world in manageable increments. Rather than being tossed onto a cold scale, the infant is gently immersed in a warm bath, reminiscent of its weightless existence in amniotic fluid. Noise and light stimulation are reduced to a minimum. The infant is supported and stroked gently rather than raised by the heels upside down and slapped. The world is slowly revealed to the infant and its response is a contented smile and, in some infants, even a laugh.

Reducing infant stress seems to pay immediate dividends in terms of its initial disposition. Whether or not long-term personality benefits accrue as well is still a topic of professional controversy, but my own guess favors Dr. Leboyer's hypothesis. I have never known stress overload to benefit anyone, and so I believe it could not benefit a fragile newborn either. Stress control methods improve everyone's ability to cope and enjoy life, and so it comes as a welcome fact that Dr. Leboyer has found that infants too appreciate the benefits of good stress control principles.

What about Dad?

So much attention has been paid to the needs of mother and infant at the time of childbirth that the other important member of the family, also undergoing major stress, has been largely forgotten. Fathers undergo a severe dislocation in their lives as a result of childbirth. Their stress arises not from physical sources, but from psychological and social ones. The father's role transition is as great as his wife's. He must assume responsibility for the life of a dependent child. He is no longer free to whisk his woman off on a carefree evening of dining and dancing. She may not have the energy, the desire, or the access to a reliable babysitter. The stresses imposed on the mother from her all-consuming moment-to-moment responsibilities for the child have direct impact on her husband as the baby's gain is his loss. He suddenly feels abandoned, the odd man out. No family or social role is clearly prescribed for him in the child's infancy stage. The baseball mitt comes later. The Barbie dolls have to wait a few years. Mother and infant are an indivisible unit, and he is merely a friendly outsider.

Men are not given a carved out role which they can rehearse prior to childbirth except to go back to work and earn lots of money to pay the hospital and obstetrician's bills.

Fathers of newborn infants go through postpartum "blues" as a result of the loss of their wife's attention and companionship.

Fathers of newborn infants are as unprepared to face the stresses of their new role and lifestyle as their newborn infants are unprepared to face the cold, noisy world of glaring lights and strange sensations.

In order to cope more effectively with the stresses of childbirth, fathers should *focus* on their task in the months to come and *rehearse* effective coping strategies. They must learn to play a new and special marital role. Because the wife is absorbed with the needs of the newborn infant, the woman's ability to cope effectively with her role as a mate is diminished. Wives who care for newborn infants are temporarily less capable social companions. Husbands must take up the slack.

The husband must become the initiator for his wife's reentry into a normal social life. He should line up a nurse, babysitter or grandmother to take charge of the infant as soon as it is feasible and begin to encourage his wife to reenter the social world and resume her other activities. He must also take a greater share of the administrative household duties to conserve his wife's energy for her draining task of caring for a demanding infant. He must become the emotional communicator in the relationship, drawing his wife's feelings to the surface and helping her accept the necessity of a temporarily more confining role. He must be there to support his wife emotionally since he cannot replace her child-rearing role with himself or anyone else.

The infant needs a contented and energetic mother. It needs a father who can help recharge mother's worn-out batteries and who can provide an emotional climate that will reassure her and lighten her spirits.

If fathers took the trouble to plan in advance how they might fulfill their new roles after the birth of their children, their stresses would be diminished, their sense of usefulness and participation would be enhanced, and their enjoyment of the entire process of childbirth would be increased.

As the recent father of a newborn, I learned to enjoy all the new duties it thrust upon me, and I even shared in the "maternal" duties of caring for the physical and emotional needs of my daughter as much as I could. I could not replace my wife's central role in the life of my infant daughter, but by sharing her duties, I could understand the joys and stresses of motherhood. I love my wife all the more for the security and contentment I see in my daughter, which has surely come about as a result of her mother's warmth and responsiveness to her. I feel personal satisfaction and a sense of achievement at having been the protective and nurturing element in my wife's life which allowed her to feel peaceful and contented while undergoing the biggest transition she will ever experience.

The way to best prepare an infant, its mother and its father for the stresses of childbirth is to apply effective stress control principles. The *quantity and pace of change must be reduced* as much as possible. *Coping skills can be increased* if both parents *focus* on their respective new roles and duties, *rehearse* these in preparation for the major changes to come, and then *implement* these stress control skills at the time of childbirth, converting that experience from an event which can run over you like a juggernaut, to a satisfying and welcome evolution.

Controlling the stresses of the childbirth transition will help you give birth comfortably not only to a new baby, but also to new roles and to a satisfying new life for each of you.

10
Sexuality and Sexual Dysfunction—A Stress Problem

Reaching The Soul through the Skin

No experience of human existence is as fragile and sensitive to the forces of stress as is that of the sexual. It is impossible to control and master sexual performance through the use of conventional coping methods since it is not subject to willpower. In fact, the more willpower used, the less satisfying and competent a person is sexually. Ordinary coping methods require you to keep your goal in sight and act in a goal-directed manner. Sexual enjoyment wilts if a performance criterion, a goal-directed action or a specific objective is kept in the center of consciousness. The woman engaging in intercourse straining to reach an elusive orgasm will never experience one. The man who promises himself that tonight he will remain hard until his wife has been masterfully and totally satisfied, will find himself unable to get it up, or to keep it up, or he will ejaculate prematurely. The stress of his trying to reach his self-imposed goal robs him of sexual vigor.

The process of engaging in satisfying sex with another person requires you to achieve three states of existence simultaneously which, when reached, will release your sexual potential without conscious effort:

1. You must be comfortable while *emotionally disrobing* with another person. In the course of lovemaking you will reveal intense feelings and so will your partner. It is essential

[163]

to be relaxed, to welcome, and to enjoy the ability to express and to witness the expression of powerful emotions. A trusting, comfortable and peaceful emotional climate must exist in the relationship as a precondition for good sex to occur.

2. You must *suspend all time considerations,* goals and performance criteria. You must live for the moment and savor sensations. The competent sexual person concentrates on smell, warmth, texture and sounds, not for orgasms and marathon lovemaking. Focus on the former and the latter will come naturally. Strive to achieve the latter without the former and you will fail.

All that counts in a satisfying sexual experience is "how I feel right now," not "how I might feel later." There is no later. There is only a boundless present, occupied by familiar sensations and the discovery of new and pleasurable feelings.

You must appreciate the level of enjoyment you have achieved. You must not compare it in your mind to a fixed criterion, such as orgasm, or the memory of another sexual experience. Otherwise, the feelings of pleasure will vanish. Sexual gratification is a primadonna feeling which is contemptuous of all other emotions and experiences. If it is not given center stage and full attention, it will leave you in a huff.

3. You must be able simultaneously to feel and *express strong aggressive feelings* as well as sexual sensations. Aggression propels the sexual act. It is made safe and guided by sexual feelings. You must trust your own and your partner's aggression and welcome it as an invigorating force in your sexual experience. Trying to restrain or eliminate the aggression within you will lead to impotence or frigidity. Trust your aggression and it will massage your sexual potential to ecstatic heights.

Two people having enjoyable sex together are engaged in a truly remarkable process. They are able to reach one another's soul through the skin. No other condition of life permits the same completeness of understanding of how another person feels at the core — at the soul of his or her existence — as does a sexual experience.

The Perpetual Discovery

Nothing destroys sexual enjoyment as easily as does stereotyped repetition. After a while, discovery must be introduced into the sexual experience or it will diminish in quality. Routine leads to boredom. Boredom is a major cause of stress. Stress is the enemy of ecstasy.

You must be experimental with sex and welcome your partner's desire to discover new sensations and experiences. You and your partner are each other's instructor and pupil simultaneously. The lesson is *pleasure*. You should teach your mate about your pleasures and then learn about those that your partner experiences. Surprise is a welcome addition to the sexual experience, if it is gently introduced.

A Case History

A couple experiencing chronic sexual problems came to my office seeking consultation in despair and frustration. They had been married fifteen years and had not had satisfactory sexual relations for most of that time.

Said the woman, "The only way he really gets turned on is when he takes me to a porno movie. Then he tries to race home and have sex. Sometimes, I swear, he tries to make it with me in the theater parking lot if nobody is around."

Her husband complained "Look, after fifteen years, sex is just sex. It's like eating tuna fish sandwiches every day for lunch for fifteen years. Unless you do something to make that tuna taste different, you lose your appetite pretty quickly."

The couple was suffering from three major problems that impaired their ability to enjoy sex:

1. They paid no attention to the emotional climate that existed between them during and prior to intercourse. Sex was seen as a goal and not as a state of physical and emotional being. They rushed, forcing themselves to perform, and consequently failed to succeed. I counseled them to limit their attempts at having sex to only those times when both partners freely desired it, no matter how infrequent this was. Liberated from the sense of obligation to satisfy the partner, each of them experienced an increase in their desire for sex.

2. They had a history of intense quarreling and attempting to make up by having sex. With the wounds of aggressive combat still raw, it was difficult for both of them to trust their own and their partner's aggression. Guilt feelings and fear dampened their aggression and consequently made sex bland and uninteresting for them. I counseled them to have sex only when they felt free of guilt and comfortable with their partner. I told them to tune into their feelings of trust and to limit their sexual experiences to times when the mood between them was peaceful, trusting and stable. They both experienced greater ease in expressing strong sexual hunger under those circumstances since they were free of guilt feelings and fear of being attacked for being greedy.

3. Their attitude toward sex was stereotyped. They regarded experimentation as perverse at worst and risky at best. "Who writes the rules for private sexual activity?" I asked. "Nobody, I guess," the wife answered. "So why do you both act as if there were a complicated set of guidelines and restrictions which confine you to one specific model of lovemaking and no other possibilities seem legal or moral to you? The only guideline in sexual experience is doing something which makes you feel good. And each of you is the judge of that for yourself." Having authorized them to experiment, they began to seek new sensations, new positions and new mental attitudes. They began to see sex as an exploration of sensations rather than a means to an end — orgasm. Their renewed enthusiasm for sex propelled them to much more pleasure than they had experienced in years. When a sexual episode failed to produce orgasm for one or

both of them, they at least felt gratified at having experienced some pleasure together instead of frustrated for having failed to reach the peak of ecstasy. As a consequence, they were more relaxed about their sexuality and finally achieved mutual orgasm much more frequently than ever before.

The advice given them followed straightforward stress control principles:

1. They *reduced* the complexity and difficulty of the task confronting them. They sought pleasurable sensations rather than reaching for orgasms and attempting to achieve a set of guidelines defining "good sex" in terms of the frequency, duration and style of the experience.
2. They *reduced* the time pressure on themselves. No deadlines were set for achieving a goal. There were no goals and no time boundaries. They got into bed together when they mutually desired to and looked forward to a pleasurable here-and-now experience. They discarded frequency and time duration criteria as stress-inducing irritants in their sexual lives.
3. They *increased* their ability to function well together by:

- *Focusing* on sensations and achieving a trusting climate between each other.
- *Rehearsing* new sexual techniques at leisure and without false restrictions.
- *Implementing* their sexual experiences with aggressive gusto, unhampered by guilt feelings and fears of attack. They felt no sense of obligation to each other or themselves and so there could be no failure. What happened happened. What didn't happen was irrelevant. They learned to enjoy sex without regret, guilt or apology.

Sexual ecstasy and stress are antagonistic properties. Only by learning to control stress will you free yourself to enjoy peak sexual experiences.

11
The Business World
and Its Stresses

Guess What Kids, We're Moving — Again

The contemporary business executive and his family have, in the last twenty years, joined the tribes of North American nomads previously consisting only of professional athletes, members of the diplomatic corps, military personnel, and, more recently, Peace Corps volunteers. Families of successful executives are often required to make successive moves on short notice on a once-every-two-years or more frequent basis. Businesses which assist transferred executives have flourished on the phenomenon of "musical cities" played by the families of corporate managers. Relocation experts promise to reduce the problems of moving to a minimum, leaving you with the simple task of exchanging the old house key for the new one and boarding a plane for a new assignment. The stresses of a relocation, however, come chiefly from sources other than having to pack your belongings and sell your house. There is a differential effect on family members exposed to a relocation, partly dependent on their personalities, partly as a function of the stage of the life cycle each member is in, and partly as a derivative of the meaning and importance of community life for each family member.

The stress points for each family member are as follows:

[169]

• Father is least affected of all. The branch of his company in Phoenix is not too different from the branch he just left in Cleveland. His work, social stimuli and rewards remain stable. The culture of his organization or industry is uniform. His major stresses that are work-related are in terms of new and greater responsibilities, or having to learn the ropes of dealing with a new boss, or with assistants, who resent his being brought in from the outside.

The major familial stresses on father are in his expanded responsibilities at home to help his family get settled, cope with his wife's loneliness until she makes new friends, and deal with his children's crankiness as they suffer homesickness and insecurity about whether they will ever be accepted by the local gang of kids.

• Mother carries an enormous burden in each relocation. Not only must she reconstruct a new home from drapes to shrubs, but she must also support her children through their readjustment trials and tribulations and, in addition, try to eke out some time to find a place for herself in the new community. If she is in a rapid personal growth phase herself when the relocation comes about, she often has to decide between impossibly unacceptable alternatives. "Do I leave my interior design course and move to Phoenix with the family, or do I tell Jim I've had enough of his job with its dislocating effects on my life? Should I tell him if he goes to Phoenix, that I'm staying here with the kids or should I once again subordinate my growth needs to his?" Mothers are hard hit by relocations and are often trapped by family loyalty into relinquishing personal growth efforts.

• Depending on their age, a move can have a different effect on each child. The rule of thumb is that the older the child, the worse the effect of the move. Younger children, up to ages six to eight, live in a world bounded by their local neighborhood and classroom. When they move, they quickly adapt to riding their bikes and playing house or cowboys and Indians in a new basement or back lawn.

The child of from nine to twelve years of age is in a stage where association with friends and participation in community activities are beginning to rival in importance the influences of home life as a means of shaping personality and social skills. Moves in this age-range disrupt this process enormously and delay or arrest the development of important ingredients of personality. The child may grow insecure, lack confidence, and retreat to more childish behavior if a move disturbs his or her first attempts at becoming accepted and recognized in the world outside the family and local neighborhood.

The teenager who is required to leave a tightly bonded group of peers, renounce a hard-won independence from the family, and move to a new community where relying on "Mom to drive me around until I know where it's at," suffers a major setback in development by relocation. Privacy and independence are essential ingredients for successful completion of teenage developmental phases. Youngsters need shelter from their parents' inquiring eyes and supervisory wisdom in order to comfortably conduct trial-and-error explorations with the new body, emotions, intellect and romantic interests suddenly acquired through their teenage metamorphosis. They do so in safety when protected by the warmth, understanding and loyalty of their peer group. Successive moves in the teenage years disrupt the stability of peer group integration and causes the teenager to cast about for other sources of privacy. Very often the teenager, searching for another sanctuary that the parents would be reluctant to invade, finds it in delinquency, the drug culture or in mental illness. The teenager needs, above all, distance from parental domination and will sacrifice safety or sanity to achieve it.

In order to cope with the stresses of relocation, parents should:

• Select proper times in the life cycle of each member in planning a relocation. Since it is impossible to synchronize life cycles in an optimum way, many times a move will cut across someone's path at an inopportune time in their development. You must assess whether that person is capable of handling a move and, if so, devote extra attention to the needs of that vulnerable family member. If a move is going to be predictably traumatic, don't do it! Delay it or the stressful consequences will exact a heavy toll. All companies who transfer executives and their families are familiar with the story of the man sent to a new assignment for a two-year period only to return in two months with a wife requiring psychiatric hospitalization and family responsibilities that hobble him in his company duties. Nobody wins in a poorly timed relocation.

• When a move is essential and feasible from a psychological point of view, it is a good practice to *focus* family interest, through a series of family discussions, on the important tasks which lie ahead. The family should *rehearse* ways of coping in the new community including, if possible, a preview trip to the new location. Little League team coaches can be met in advance. Girl Scout leaders will be pleased to meet a new girl several months before the move. A stroll through the new shopping center and park will reveal many familiar and reassuring sights. *Reduce* the amount of change that has to be dealt with by making the move in installments — mind first, belongings next. Make the transition as gradual as possible. *Reducing* time pressure by having as much advance notice as possible will significantly lower the stress of the move.

The Stress of Promotion

The fortunate employee who receives a sought after promotion will surely get more than he or she bargained for. It is in our nature to expect that "the grass is always greener one level above where I am." I have found in my own career that I was always happier at the lower level than when I assumed the top position myself.

There are successively *less* rather than *more* degrees of freedom with every move you make up the ladder. Because of your increased responsibility, you make creative changes less freely at the top than you would have lower down the hierarchy. All eyes are on you and ready to criticize you if you goof. You are *more* accountable at the top of an organization than at the bottom. Payoffs come less rapidly to the boss than to his subordinates. The employee on the assembly line sees the cars he has constructed roll off the line several times a day; he picks up his paycheck at the end of the week and goes home to enjoy his wife, family and community.

His boss is busy making five-year projections that may or may not prove sound — only time will tell. He must carry his work home evenings and on the weekends. His wife becomes an "asset" to further his career rather than a person in her own right to be enjoyed. Moving up the ladder tightens the stress bonds around your freedom to live as you want to — it forces you to consider the company's needs above your own and those of your family.

You deserve the raise you got with your last paycheck. What you didn't see was the amount of your freedom deducted at the source.

The stresses of a promotion must be weighed against the needs you yourself have and your family's needs for you. Before you trade a piece of your freedom, time and peace of mind for more money, make sure you and your family evaluate which is more important to you. I have known many executives who cleverly duck the top spot for many years, being content to remain in the number two position. They trade status and a few thousand dollars for a significantly better lifestyle and never regret their choice.

Those Who Travel and Their Spouses

As more and more women move up the managerial ladder, they experience the same stresses as male executives — including those imposed by travel. The effects on marital relationships are, naturally, essentially the same — or possible *more* stressful, as many men have yet to cope effectively with having a wife who is as career-oriented as they are.

Aside from the obvious loss of time together experienced by the traveling executive and his or her mate, two major stresses occur which can be significant:

1. The loss of control over the other person's life can be experienced as a threat or destabilizing force in the relationship. "What if she finds someone else to love in her travels? What if absence makes the ties grow weaker rather than the heart grow fonder?" The traveling executive has similar fears. "She could be home carrying on while I'm stuck in this sixteen-dollar-a-night motel," he fumes.

Many relationships are founded on the mistaken belief that, "My partner acts the way he/she does because I'm there to supervise. When I turn my back, watch out!" Living with another person gives us a false belief that somehow our own will can permeate the other person by osmosis and influence or even control their behavior.

The fact is that your partner shares your life because it is in his or her best interest to do so. You fill needs, you provide stability, comfort, and peace of mind. Try to replace these with remote control, and you will have to really watch out. "Phone me every evening or give me your number so that I can phone you" is often a phrase that conveys so much mistrust that the comforts of home are not remembered by the traveler. Instead, he looks forward to "getting the phone call over with so that I can get down to the bar, have a few drinks and see who's there."

Don't pretend to yourself or to your spouse that you can control his or her behavior either up close or at a distance of hundreds of miles. If you talk by phone, remember that your spouse needs you for comfort and stability. Reassurance and empathy will bring forth more loyalty than suspicion.

2. Abandonment is the most primitive and powerful fear anyone can experience. We all have had different

experiences with respect to abandonment in our growing up years, and, consequently, our abilities to handle the stresses of temporary abandonment are of different strengths.

As a young child, I was hospitalized several times for serious illnesses. I have a built-in allergy to abandonment that years of psychoanalysis and all the logic in the world can't cure. Since I am always going to have a vulnerability to abandonment, I can only make the best of the situation. Temporary separations cannot be avoided but their impact can be reduced. I take several short rather than one long business trip if possible and feasible. I minimize my feelings of loneliness by setting up social engagements when on business trips. Where possible, I take my wife along. I'm not shy about my allergy to abandonment, but I have reduced its stressful impact on me through careful planning and by reducing the amount of loneliness I must deal with at any one time.

Retirement Stresses

Tell an employee reaching retirement age that he is lucky to soon be able to live for himself and soak up the sun, and he will internally cringe. Memories — too fresh to ignore — of recent retirees' funerals remind him that the long awaited life of leisure may turn out to have some hidden stresses that can be and often are *fatal*.

If you consider that the magnitude of any change determines the amount of stress it produces, then retirement is one of the most stressful times of all of life. Consider these aspects of retirement:

- Hard-won job status is relinquished the day your retirement takes effect.
- You give up looking forward to a future and are told it is important for you to enjoy the present. "How do I do this?" you puzzle. "I've never had so much time on my hands

since I was a preschooler." Understimulation produces as much stress as overstimulation and the retired employee, unprepared for leisure, is under major stress due to the loss of all stimulation previously afforded by the job.

• "How do we cope with each other twenty-four hours a day?" complains the retired couple who suddenly spend more time together in one day of retirement than they had with each other in many a week of their previous life.

• Social isolation is felt suddenly as "all the guys are still at the office and I'm stuck here in a condominium in the sun with few people I know or care to meet."

• The long-forgotten skill of introspection is spontaneously revived, and the retiree is disturbed by long-suppressed thoughts and fears. "How long will my sexual potency last? Will inflation curb my lifestyle? When will death come?"

The retirement stage is better handled if you employ good stress control principles. A *reduction* in the proportions of the stress is possible if the person phases out of work and phases into leisure over a period of several years. This gives the person a chance to establish a new life pattern without *time pressure* and in small installments. Consider the case of Tom, a senior employee who came in for counseling to the STRESSCONTROL Center.

"I can't fault them at the company. They probably saved my life when I had a heart attack two years ago. Besides giving me a generous medical leave with pay, they rallied around me like the loyal friends I've known them to be for the past twenty-five years. When I got back to work the boss had tears in his eyes when he told me that my job function was taken over by my assistant. I ended up consoling him. After all, the company's well-being shouldn't depend on a sixty-four-year-old heart — a scarred one at that." Tom spoke like the dedicated company man he had been for years and then got down to the reason for his visit to the STRESSCONTROL Center.

"I haven't been sleeping well at all. I think I'm depressed. This illness really drove home the fact I've been trying to avoid for years. The big days for me are over. Retirement is coming up in a few months, and I feel under more pressure now than ever before. The kids want me to move in with them. They're afraid I'll be lonely. I've gotten on well since Emily passed away but, without the job, maybe I would be too isolated. Yet I hate to be a burden to them. They have their own lives to lead."

Tom had many problems to face in the coming months. He would encounter these major turning points in his life, initiated by the single act of retiring:

- Should I remain independent and combat loneliness myself, or should I move in with my children?
- Are my savings adequate to sustain long-term independent living, or would it be economically wiser to swallow my pride and become more financially dependent on my children?
- What will I do to fill all the empty time?
- How will I combat the depression caused by being out of harness, feeling like extra baggage wherever I go?
- My health is a big concern. What do I do to maintain it?

The stresses of retirement are many and are serious. If a retirement is unplanned, all these stresses must be dealt with concurrently, which can be overwhelming. Tom was counseled to reduce the number of tasks he was trying to solve. Take on only the most immediate ones and then deal with the rest in order of priority. Most pressing for Tom was the need for good social and financial counseling. Tom was put in touch with a senior citizens community action and resource center. Through their fund of information he was able to select and pursue many avenues to keep him socially and intellectually stimulated. He chose to explore some adult education courses at the community college; he enrolled in a senior citizens political action group; he began setting up a home workshop since he had always been an inventor but never had the time to develop his ideas. Through these activities he met a large number of retired men and women with whom he began to socialize. In fact, he could hardly wait for his retirement date in some respects, since the enthusiasm he shared with members of the senior citizens political action group was invigorating and had real significance for him as compared with the meaningless work assigned to him since his heart attack.

His financial counselor showed him how to shave his cost of living and boost the interest brought in by his savings. He realized that he had adequate funds for independent living with enough reserve for travel as well.

We counseled him to reduce the time pressures on himself for decision making. We advised him to defer his decision about where to live for one to two years. He decided to have a trial period of independent living. If he was still uncertain, he would then try out a period of living with his children. After comparing these two experiences, he would be able to decide more adequately what to do, rather than rushing blindly into a dependency on his children out of fear of loneliness.

We encouraged Tom to structure his life. Not having a job doesn't mean that one should abandon planning and scheduling one's activities. Too much time on your hands can be as much of a pressure as not enough time. Tom set out a daily and weekly schedule of activities and tasks and found that this method helped him make a smooth transition between work and retirement.

Tom was told which physical functions might fade with increasing age and what to do about them when that happened. He was encouraged to exercise, avoid overeating and continue his practice of having annual physical exams.

Tom had always had a desire to travel to the Far East and now he had the time and money to do so. He feared the possibility of falling ill in a foreign country and not knowing how to find a qualified English-speaking doctor. We advised him to subscribe to an excellent publication called *Intermedic,* which lists qualified doctors all over the world who speak English. Thus reassured, he made plans for a trip to the Orient.

Tom's retirement dilemma was typical of most we encounter. Retirement is stressful, lonely and full of decisions for which an individual feels inadequately prepared and poorly informed.

Coping methods during retirement can be improved if the person is psychologically prepared for the transition. At the STRESSCONTROL Center, we conduct seminars for executives several years before their retirement age. We help them *focus* on the tasks and rehearse solutions to the stresses they will face upon retirement: their loneliness and their need to resocialize; their need to replace job status with other ego-building pursuits; their need for stimulation and activity; how to handle the renewed and intensified husband-wife relationship; the new opportunities for reflection and how these can be used productively; caring for one's health in the senior years.

Retirement can be a death sentence for a vigorous person if its stresses are not controlled. If the company and individual take pains to effect a smooth, unhurried and stress controlled transition, retirement will be a stimulating and enviable period of self-renewal that is much deserved as a reward for years of hard work and loyalty.

12
Stress Control in Everyday Living

Taking Stock of Stress

Someone once said to me, "Money is unimportant. It is the *absence* of money that is important." The same can be said of stress control. When things are going well, we pay little attention to our state of mind and to our health. The moment stress gets out of hand, we become urgently aware of the importance of controlling stress. Try to ignore a migraine headache or a heart which persists in palpitating — both stress overload manifestations. You can't. When stress control has not been practiced, the price in physical and/or emotional discomfort can be very high.

It is a far wiser and more productive use of your energy, time and effort if you regularly apply stress control principles in the course of daily living to *avoid stress overload* rather than to *repair its consequences*. You practice preventive maintenance if you own a stereo, automobile, airplane or home. You buy magazines on the care and handling of your stereo. You monitor your car's well-being in advance of trouble, regularly checking the oil, battery fluid, antifreeze level, and tire tread depth. Apply the same kind of daily care and attention to the stresses in your life and you will live longer and with more peace of mind.

You must develop a *checklist for stress overload* symptoms. Each person has a particular pattern of reactions to stress which can be used as a barometer or early warning system to indicate when stress is approaching overload levels. The following listing will help you construct your **Stress Profile:**

Social Sphere
1. Too much change going on in my life (See the Holmes and Rahe checklist of life events in Chapter 1.)
2. Repeated problems with people at work
3. Recurrent marital problems
4. Family conflicts that cannot be resolved
5. Inadequate number of friends and confidants

The Mind
1. Inability to shut down thought processes; insomnia
2. Chronic difficulties with memory
3. Distractability
4. Chronic procrastination and ambivalence

The Emotions
1. All emotions feel too intense.
2. It takes very little to set me off.
3. I can't get unstuck from one particular emotion.
4. I don't react when and how I should. I don't feel emotions the way other people do.

The Body
1. I have destructive habits such as nail biting, grinding my teeth, picking at sores and not letting them heal, etc.
2. I eat, drink and/or use medications to excess.
3. I suffer from recurrent headaches.
4. I hear "head noises" or "ringing in my ears" and my doctor says there is nothing physically wrong with me.
5. I suffer from chronic eye strain.
6. I periodically feel that I can't get enough air into my lungs to satisfy me and yet my doctor says I am healthy.
7. I have palpitations and my doctor says my heart is O.K.
8. My blood pressure fluctuates widely. The doctor has to take it several times before getting a normal reading.

9. I have an acid stomach.
10. I constantly am gassy; I burp a lot.
11. I have diarrhea frequently and yet my doctor says my health is good and it's probably due to "nerves."
12. I seem to need to urinate more frequently than normal and yet my doctor tells me I'm not diabetic, have no kidney or bladder problems, or any other type of disease.
13. I get muscle cramps, stiff necks and backaches frequently.
14. My hands tremble.
15. I seem to have a low pain threshold.
16. My hands and/or feet often get cold and sweaty.
17. My skin is excessively oily.
18. My face flushes often.

Out of the above list, you will be able to select those specific social, mental, emotional, and physical symptoms which constitute your **Stress Profile,** your unique way of reacting to stress. Now you must learn to detect these manifestations as soon as they become evident and associate them with what is going on in your life at that moment. In that way, you will be able to analyze your daily life in terms of the events that cause stress overload.

By further examining the way you live, you can assess whether you have adequate social supports and outlets; whether your creative-esthetic needs are being satisfied; whether your diet is balanced and nutritious; and whether you engage in a regular and sufficient amount of physical exercise.

Glance at the Health Promoting Flow System chart on the next page and you will be able to put together a specific **Stress Control Plan** that matches your needs as revealed by your **Stress Profile.** Each discrete factor on the flow chart should be reviewed and a stress control plan developed to improve your ability to function in each area.

A HEALTH-PROMOTING FLOW SYSTEM

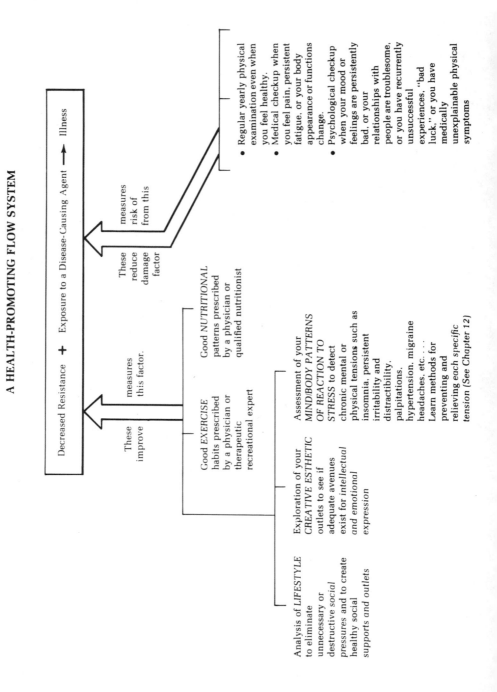

Decreased Resistance **+** Exposure to a Disease-Causing Agent → Illness

These improve

These reduce damage factor

measures this factor.

measures risk of from this

Good NUTRITIONAL patterns prescribed by a physician or qualified nutritionist

Good EXERCISE habits prescribed by a physician or therapeutic recreational expert

Assessment of your MIND/BODY PATTERNS OF REACTION TO STRESS to detect chronic mental or physical tensions such as insomnia, persistent irritability and distractibility, palpitations, hypertension, migraine headaches, etc. . . . Learn methods for preventing and relieving each specific tension (See Chapter 12)

Exploration of your CREATIVE ESTHETIC outlets to see if adequate avenues exist for intellectual and emotional expression

Analysis of LIFESTYLE to eliminate unnecessary or destructive social pressures and to create healthy social supports and outlets

- Regular yearly physical examination even when you feel healthy.
- Medical checkup when you feel pain, persistent fatigue, or your body appearance or functions change.
- Psychological checkup when your mood or feelings are persistently bad, or your relationships with people are troublesome, or you have recurrently unsuccessful experiences, "bad luck," or you have medically unexplainable physical symptoms

Unstressing Your Mind

The essence of a good **Stress Control Plan** is a reprogramming of your mind's and body's responses to stress.

This is the unhealthy pattern of stress response:

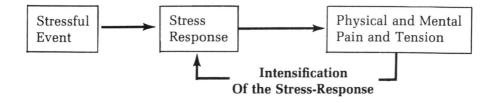

A self-intensifying cycle is established in response to a stressful event and it leads ultimately to destructive stress overload. We must learn to reprogram the mind and body responses to stress as follows:

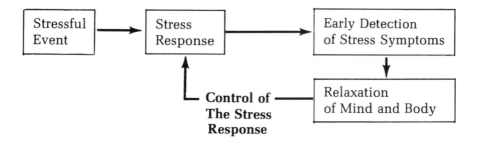

There are three useful methods of relaxing your mind:

1. Learning to reduce the complexity and number of tasks that confront you helps to reduce stress. You cope more effectively when problems are handled one-by-one on a priority system and in manageable installments.
2. Learning to reduce the time pressure on yourself helps to reduce stress. Nature has been good to us by giving us a natural reflex of reducing time pressure when faced by overwhelming stress.

Recently, my seventeen-month-old daughter got into a bottle of her grandfather's heart medication and swallowed a large quantity of pills. When notified, I rushed over to the emergency room and remained with her throughout the crisis. My time focus was reduced to a span of no more than five minutes at a time. "How do I keep her alive? Will I be able to get her to vomit up the pills? What do I do about her irregular pulse? Will she be alive five minutes from now?" My mind narrowed down to immediate issues. Had a colleague strolled by and said, "Hi, did you hear about the important staff meeting tomorrow?" I would have shut him quickly out of my consciousness. There was no room in my mind for more than one five-minute slice of life at a time.

Regrettably, many of us fight nature's automatic mental stress control mechanism. When under pressure, some people rush, and look down the road too far to distant goals. The business executive who is under stress in coping with his current staff morale problems may begin to worry about "what this might do to my reputation and to my ultimate career goals." Rather than projecting into the future, he would be best off to cope with the problem at hand. Otherwise, in trying to dispose of the problem too quickly, and distracted by worries about the future, he could impose excessive stress on himself which would undermine rather than facilitate his ability to cope with the situation. Make time work for you in order to reduce stress. Use it to set a comfortable pace for coping with problems. Don't beat yourself up with an arbitrary time schedule that works against your own success.

3. Mind-focusing exercises are very helpful ways of reducing mental stress. Various meditative methods have been developed and promoted to help people unload tensions by focusing their mind on neutral thoughts — such as a mantra, or a number, or deep breathing. The mind, which is able to remain attached to neutral mental processes, is capable of temporarily escaping from stress. In effect, meditation allows you to put your mental burdens down several times per day, rest your mind for twenty minutes, and then pick your burdens up again with more mental energy.

I train myself to focus by periodically visualizing my mind as a fish tank. If you want to study a particular fish in a home aquarium, you track that fish with your eyes wherever it swims in the tank. When other fish swim through your field of vision, you are aware of their presence but you don't follow their track. You may be momentarily distracted from your study of the selected fish by another fish in the tank, but you return your attention as quickly as possible to the object of your study despite the intrusion.

Your thoughts, body sensations, and the distractions surrounding you are all like fish in your mental aquarium. You can train yourself through daily practice to attend to one thought or one body sensation and not be drawn away by the other stimuli which may, from moment-to-moment, float through your conscious mind.

It has been found that people who practice mind-focusing or meditation respond better to stress. They seem to recover much more rapidly from the effects of stress than non-meditators.*

*Daniel J. Goleman and Gary E. Schwartz, "Meditation as an Intervention in Stress Reactivity," JOURNAL OF CONSULTING AND CLINICAL PSYCHOLOGY, Vol. 44. no. 3 (1976), 456–466

Unstressing Your Emotions

The stress control sequence that should be set into action by an emotion is as follows:

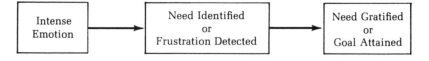

Very often, this sequence is unproductively interfered with in several ways:

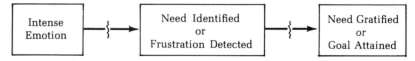

1. Failure to use the emotion as a signal to initiate a search for important unfulfilled needs.

2. Needs detected but the information is discarded without examination.

1. Fear of satisfying need because it would be too greedy or assertive to do so.

2. Excessively rigid standards and un- workable values prohibit need gratification.

3. Goals are set at too difficult a level, producing constant failure resulting in pessimism and with- drawal.

4. No goals are clearly established for satisfying needs.

5. Person waits for comfort to precede mastery rather than the reverse. Consequently, the time is never ripe to initiate a solution.

When an individual permits these interferences in the need-gratifying process of daily life, emotional stress will grow to overload proportions. You can overcome emotional stress by applying the stress control formula as follows:

- *Focus* on the need underlying the emotion.
- *Rehearse* mentally a positive solution for satisfying your need.
- *Implement* that solution. If your values or standards interfere with need satisfaction, they may need revision. You must set clear, attainable goals for need satisfaction. You should realize that comfort comes after mastery and not before. Solving problems and making necessary changes is stressful and uncomfortable. Accepting the small doses of stress and discomfort which accompany change helps to avoid much greater stress that can result from chronically unfulfilled needs and painful, inescapable emotions.

Unstressing Your Body

The body's response to stress is highly complex and varied according to the individual affected. Some of us react to stress with stomach upset, others with cold, clammy hands, still others with labored breathing. The list of physical discomforts produced by stress is long. The way to reduce physical stress is relatively simple.

The principle underlying physical stress control is that it is impossible for anyone to exist in two contradictory states simultaneously. You can't be short and tall at the same time. You can't be pregnant and not pregnant concurrently. Vigor and fatigue cannot coexist. Similarly, it is impossible to be stressed and physically relaxed at the same time. If you know how to find the state of physical relaxation and how to sustain it, you will be better able to prevent the occurrence of physical stress overload and will be able to control excessive tension once it has occurred.

The stress control formula is once again useful here. You need to learn how to *focus* on physically relaxed states; how to *rehearse* physical relaxation responses until they can be achieved quickly and with ease; and then learn when and how to *implement* the physical relaxation response at a time preceding or during a stressful event.

Focusing on a physically relaxed state is achieved by three means:

1. *Diaphragmatic breathing* in slow, four-second "in," and four-second "out" excursions, assists the relaxation process. Lie down on a flat surface, facing up. Place your hand on your stomach. When you breathe in, your stomach should slowly rise because the diaphragm, acting like a piston, moves out of the chest cavity to suck air into your lungs. At the same time, the diaphram descends into the abdominal cavity, pushing your intestines down and forward — the cause of your rising stomach. Exhale slowly and your stomach falls. Your rib cage should be quite still. It is only needed during extreme exertion. Breathing to a count of four on each inhalation and exhalation is a restful breathing pattern.

2. Next, you must learn to relax your muscles and blood vessels. When your blood vessels are relaxed, your hands feel warm. When the blood vessels in your body are tense, your hands feel cold and clammy. You can increase the warmth of your hands by focusing on the sensations in your hand as it rests on the arm of the chair beside you. I'm sure you feel sensations of touch. You can feel the texture of the arm of the chair upon which your hand rests. Whatever the room temperature may be, your hands can feel both the sensations of airy coolness as well as warmth. If you wish to intensify the warmth, simply keep "warmth" in a relaxed focus in your mind. Imagine lying on a sunny beach with the sun beating down on your hand. Imagine your body filling up with warmth from the toes on up.

To relax your muscles, you can take the hand that is gently resting on the arm of the chair beside you and tense all your fingers without pressing them into the chair. Your hand will feel like it is hovering just above the arm of the chair. Tense muscles make your limbs feel *light*. Now relax your arm, wrist, and fingers. The limb feels *heavy* as it slouches on the arm of the chair.

Now, starting from the top of your head, proceeding through every muscle and joint in your body down to your toes, contract each muscle to feel the sensation of tension — the lightness — and then feel the weight and heaviness associated with muscular relaxation.

You must now learn to *rehearse* warming your hands, relaxing your muscles and joints, and breathing slowly with your diaphragm. Take twenty minutes to do so. Don't watch the clock. Just guess at a time span of roughly twenty minutes and rehearse the relaxation of your breathing, blood vessels and muscles.

While relaxing your body, you may wish to simultaneously relax your mind using a mind-focusing exercise, as described above. When I practice relaxation, I breathe in cycles of three breaths repeating in my mind:

Breath # 1 — "Give up caring"
Breath # 2 — "Heavy and warm"
Breath # 3 — "Breathe and relax"

As distractions enter my consciousness, I don't let them trouble me, even if they temporarily throw me off my pattern. I simply resume my slow, three-breath cycle of:

Breath # 1 — "Give up caring"
Breath # 2 — "Heavy and warm"
Breath # 3 — "Breathe and relax"

When you have *rehearsed* these relaxation exercises for a period of several days, you can then begin to implement them in your daily life.

I do this for myself in two ways:

1. Whenever I think about *stress*, or *relaxation*, or a future *problem* or anything else even remotely associated with stress, I begin to relax in the manner outlined above. The reason for this is that I want to reinforce the new "program" in my physical system for controlling stress. I want to condition myself to automatically and invariably respond to stress, in all its manifestations, by a relaxation of physical tension. I think to myself, "It's not necessary to beat myself up physically just because the guy in that car cut me off; or why should I get a stiff neck or back just because my boss is in a bad mood."

If a full relaxation exercise is not feasible at the time, I do as much relaxing as circumstances permit. A while back I was flying through a heavy rainstorm with severe turbulence. I let my right arm and hand dangle by my side on the seat and warmed and relaxed that limb. My whole body responded in a more relaxed way even though it was only possible to actually free up one limb for direct relaxation. You can practice this type of partial relaxation as I do, unnoticed, in the course of driving your car, or in a business meeting, or between rallies on a tennis court. You will not lose mental alertness and will be physically less tense, less fatigued and more energetic.

2. Regularly scheduled daily relaxation practice will improve your state of physical and mental well-being and also will reinforce the reprogramming of your mind and body towards healthier stress responses. Twenty minutes of relaxation practice just before falling asleep will suffice for this type of training and will also help you fall asleep more quickly and easily.

Throughout this book, I have emphasized the principles of stress control. It is not possible or desirable to eliminate stress from life. Stress is an essential ingredient of life, preparing you to cope with emergencies that arise. Without the stress response to mobilize needed resources quickly, you would succumb to any mental, emotional or physical challenge of consequence. The purpose of stress control methods is to *demobilize* the *stress response as soon as it is not needed*, returning your body and mind to a *harmonious and normal state* so as to conserve energy for any subsequent emergencies. Practicing stress control methods will enable you to acquire mental, emotional, and physical tranquility as an enduring and attainable basis for daily living.

Appendix:
Biofeedback

What is Biofeedback?

The human body is operated by two master control systems. One is under voluntary conscious control, as the movements that guide your eyes across this page. You can direct your eyes at will to any point on the page. The other system operates automatically, like the dilation and contraction of your pupils in dark or light surroundings. Some body functions utilize both systems, like eye-blinking or breathing. These functions proceed rhythmically and reflexively but can be brought under conscious control at will.

Stress affects both these body systems, causing excessive and persistent activity that can be damaging to health. Migraine sufferers know the severe consequences stress can produce when blood vessels silently and automatically contract all over the body, starving the brain of needed blood flow. People suffering from palpitations experience extreme fears of dying. Their excessively rapid heartbeats are propelled by an unremitting stress reaction.

Since stress operates as a *silent alarm*, these body systems are called into action without warning and can build up a fierce momentum, undetectable by an untrained person until severe

[195]

stress symptoms surface. At this point, stress is out of control and is potentially dangerous to health.

Biofeedback is a process by which electronic devices are used to tune into your body's stress reactions. These instruments are so sensitive that they can detect even minute quantities of stress. As this stress information is electronically sensed, it is transformed into a signal: either an audible tone, a light signal or a deviation on a meter dial. You are immediately alerted to the inner workings of your stress reactions through these signals and are now in a position to learn how to detect and control stress before it reaches dangerous levels.

This learning process is similar to the way in which a child learns how to control and coordinate the movement of his or her hand. At first the infant needs to look at the function of the hand in order for there to be coordinated movement. The child moves the hand, waves the hand, bangs it against something and visually observes the reaction of the object (for example a rattle) to the movement of the hand. After a while, the child's hand can operate in a coordinated fashion without the visual feedback. The child is able to manipulate objects without direct visualization — that is, without visual feedback. Eventually, hand movement becomes second nature to the child and no thought or feedback is necessary for smoothly coordinated hand activity.

Similarly, an individual learning biofeedback relaxation methods can learn to develop voluntary control over specific functions that are causing problems — for example, a person with migraine headaches can learn to control blood vessel dilation and thus abort an impending migraine headache. People who tend to be chronically anxious can learn to use a combination of relaxation techniques to reduce anxiety and tension. Many other conditions respond favorably to biofeedback relaxation therapy including:

- insominia
- psychosomatic illnesses
- bruxism (teeth grinding)
- tinnitus (ringing in the ears)
- fluctuating high blood pressure

- palpitations
- angina
- muscle cramps and backaches

How Do I Learn Biofeedback Relaxation Techniques?

Using the stress control formula outlined in this book, you learn to focus on body functions through the use of biofeedback equipment; then you rehearse relaxation techniques (a combination of mental and physical exercises) that reduce the unnecessary mobilization of body systems in response to stress; finally, you learn how to implement these techniques in the course of your daily life:

- Biofeedback relaxation techniques can only work if they are *practiced and then applied when stressful situations occur.*
- Biofeedback relaxation techniques are *safe* and cannot be overdone. You may use these important stress control methods anytime you feel discomfort, or in order to tune up for an important meeting or tennis match.
- Biofeedback relaxation methods are meant to *recondition your body reflexes* so that you can learn to sense and control stress before it gets out of hand. The equipment used is a learning aid and can quickly be dispensed with as soon as you learn to tune in to your body's stress reactions. Usually, five to fifteen hours of training suffices for this to be accomplished.
- No amount of biofeedback training will reverse existing bodily damage produced by stress. Biofeedback is a *preventive technique.* Consequently, it *should be used by healthy people* and also by those who suffer from *reversible stress-induced illnesses* such as labile hypertension, migraine, Raynaud's disease, angina pectoris, to name only a few. People with definite pathological changes in their

organs may benefit from biofeedback but in these cases, the biofeedback therapy should be under the close medical supervision of a qualified physician.

Are There Any Dangers in the Professional Use of Biofeedback?

Biofeedback equipment is an outgrowth of space-age technology. It uses very sophisticated electronic methods to monitor bodily processes. Biofeedback instruments are battery operated and are totally passive so that no electrical energy passes from the instrument to the body. They only monitor body activity.

Can I Become Dependent on the Equipment and Need It as a Crutch?

With respect to dependency on the equipment, good techniques emphasize using the biofeedback equipment only to assist the learning process. In a relatively short period of time a learning situation evolves in which one becomes conscious of involuntary functions, such as body temperature, muscle activity, etc. Soon after that, the biofeedback equipment equipment can be dispensed with and an individual retains voluntary control over these previously involuntary functions.

Do I Have to be Sick to Benefit from Biofeedback Relaxation Training?

More and more, biofeedback relaxation training is being used by a very wide range of individuals who wish to reduce the chances of being adversely affected by the stresses and strains of modern-day life. Just as a thermostat can be set to a desired temperature, it is possible through biofeedback relaxation training to set the body's physiological responses to stress at an optimum level. There is quite good evidence available currently that this acquired ability significantly improves the individual's feelings of well-being and resistance to the destructive potential of stress, chronic anxiety, and so on. In this sense, its greatest promise is as a preventive technique for use by healthy people under stress who wish to optimize their functioning.

How Can I Select a Good Biofeedback Program for Myself?

So far, there is no accepted national standard to qualify people as biofeedback experts. Consequently, many people have entered the field with dollars in hand to establish impressive looking "clinics," and with a motivation for profit that far exceeds their know-how. Some tips may be helpful in selecting a good program:

1. If the institution offering the program is a government regulated and certified one, then the biofeedback program meets professional standards.
2. If a private therapist or clinic offers biofeedback, make sure that the program is supervised by a certified or licensed psychologist or a qualified physician.
3. Ask these questions before entering the training program:
— How long have you been doing biofeedback?
— What is your success rate with my condition?
— May I call one or two of your clients who have completed their training to ask about their results and satisfaction?
— Can you tell me where you learned to do biofeedback? Is it all right if I call that person or institution to verify your credentials?

Ordinarily, a competent biofeedback therapist will not hesitate to answer these questions in a helpful way. After all, we know that the field is new and people have a right to be curious and even skeptical.

Index